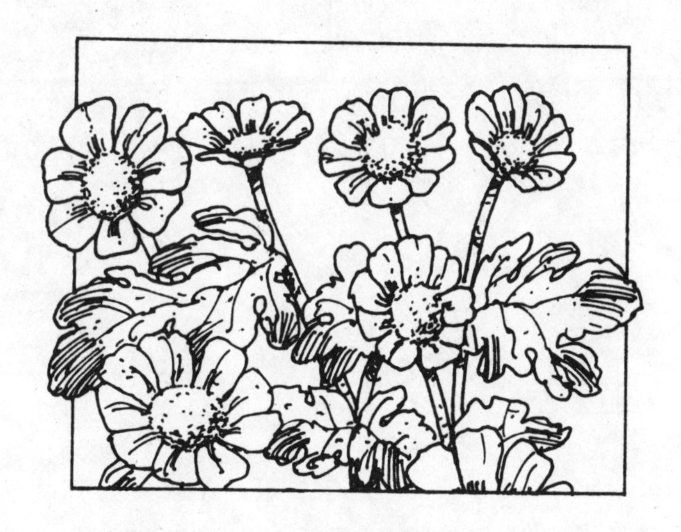

FEVERFEW

YOUR HEADACHE MAY BE OVER

AUTHOR'S NOTE

The information contained in this book is presented only as a general educational and informational guide. It is not intended as medical advice. Treatment of illness, including any condition which appears to be related to migraine should be treated and supervised by a physician or other appropriate and licensed health professional. This book is not intended as advice for self-diagnosis. For obvious reasons, neither the author or the publisher can assume the medical or legal responsibility of having the contents of this book misinterpreted and considered as a prescription for any condition or any person.

FEVERFEW

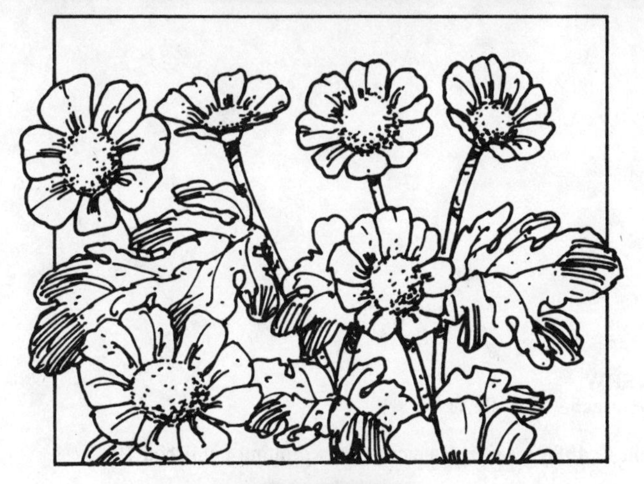

YOUR HEADACHE MAY BE OVER

Ken Hancock

Introduction by William H. Lee, R.Ph., Ph.D.
author of *Herbs and Herbal Medicine*
Preface by Paul Lee, Ph.D.
With a note on the botany and pharmacology of Feverfew by Christopher Hobbs, Herbalist

Keats Publishing, Inc. New Canaan, Connecticut

FEVERFEW
Your Headache May Be Over

Library of Congress Cataloging-in-Publication Data
Hancock, Ken.
The feverfew story.

1. Feverfew—Therapeutic use. I. Hobbs, Christopher. Note on the botany and pharmacology of feverfew. 1986. II. Title.
RM666.F44H36 1986 615'.32'355 85-63479
ISBM 0-87983-392-0

Printed in the United States of America

Published by Keats Publishing, Inc.
27 Pine Street (Box 876)
New Canaan, Connecticut 06840

Contents

DEDICATION

This book is dedicated to Gladys and Vao Cheney
of San Leandro, California,
with my thanks to a lovely couple.

ACKNOWLEDGMENTS

I gratefully acknowledge the help I have received from friends, neighbours and relatives. There were times when I received thousands of enquiries within a short space of time due to the publication of letters in newspapers; and without their assistance, the replies would have taken so much longer.

I thank my wife, too, for she has worked long and hard for the cause of Feverfew, in the full knowledge that she could not derive benefit from the herb. She has put up with long lonely hours while I have been engaged with the research.

My thanks are also due to Jack and Kathy Turner, who have given unstintingly of their time in providing a postal service from their small health food shop. This was a major problem for me, for at one time, I was receiving hundreds of letters asking for location of supplies. Jack and Kathy provided this service at nothing above cost, although it involved a great deal of extra work. It still makes extra work for them because many customers have become close pen-pals, and the number is growing. They will retire soon, but they have no intention of deserting Feverfew.

When you have read through this book—carefully, I hope—and you have a question to which you cannot find an answer, write to me at 80, Holbrook Road, Alvaston, Derby DE20DF, England, and I will be pleased to help if I can. Please enclose a stamped, self-addressed envelope because I fund my own research, and the number of enquiries is increasing all the time. One other thing, don't try to telephone because the number is unlisted; before this was so, it was ringing from 0600 to well past midnight.

I do want to hear from you about your experience with the herb, whether it is good, bad or indifferent. As you will see, the area of involvement of the herb is spreading, and your experience could be responsible for cracking wide open another avenue of research, helping thousands, perhaps millions, of sufferers.

Best wishes

Ken Hancock

INTRODUCTION

by William H. Lee, R.Ph., Ph.D.

Migraine headaches have no respect for celebrities or national boundries. Sigmund Freud, Virginia Woolf, Thomas Jefferson, Ulysses S. Grant and millions of Americans, Russians, Swedes, Italians, and others were and are unlucky enough to be "migraineurs."

Migraine victims seem to inherit a biochemistry that is unusually vulnerable, a blood vessel system that is easily dilated by emotional stress as well as changes in air pressure, odors, temperature, type A behavior, sleep deprivation and other more-or-less normal factors. When it strikes, the torturing head pains can continue for hours or even days before releasing its paralyzing hold.

Physicians have used ergotamine tartrate alone or in combination with caffeine as a treatment for migraine but frequently the treatment becomes addictive which, in turn, triggers off more attacks. Also, long-term daily use of painkillers—codeine, demerol, aspirin and acetaminophen—may actually make the throbbing worse.

For these, and other reasons, the author of this book deserves a thank you for offering to the American people an opportunity to become acquainted with an old herbal remedy *Tanacetum parthenium*, also known as *Feverfew*.

Although known for centuries as the best cure for the worst headaches, it was not until 1980 that serious attempts to understand its pharmacology and activity were undertaken in England, and even now, if it were not for the efforts of the author, Ken Hancock, it would have remained an obscure British treatment.

Mr. Hancock does not have an overpowering style of writing. His book is more anecdotal than filled with references to double-blind studies (although many have been done and published. You can refer to *The Lancet*, October 25, 1980, also *The Lancet* November 7, 1981, and the *British Medical Journal* Volume 291, August 31, 1985).

The letters he has received and published present a native response to the pleasure of discovering a natural substance that actually works for them. The facts speak more powerfully from these works than if the author was more eloquent in his presentation.

He says he has not written the book to get you to rush out to the nearest shop to purchase some Feverfew tablets or capsules, or to plant the shrub in your garden or windowbox. What he has attempted to do is to give you the whole picture, not only as he has seen it, but as it is through the eyes of so many people qualified by experience of Feverfew as well as the many synthetic drugs they've tried during their years of suffering.

The letters describe the relief felt not only from migraine conditions but also in other conditions including certain arthritic inflammations. Interestingly enough, Queen's medical Center, Nottingham, England, upon investigating the activity of Feverfew, discovered that an extract of the leaf was capable of inhibiting PMNS (polymorphonuclear leucocytes) which have a damaging effect on inflamed joints and skin.

When the *British Medical Journal* ran an article relating to the efficacy of Feverfew as prophylactic treatment of migraine, the introduction stated that the plant was a medicinal herb commonly used in self-treatment for conditions such as migraine and arthritis. They continued that in one survey more than 70% of 270 migraine sufferers who had eaten Feverfew leaves every day for prolonged periods claimed that the herb decreased the frequency of the attacks or caused them to be less painful, or both.

Many of these people have failed to respond to orthodox medicine.

There are many good herbal remedies around. This book reveals one of the best of them.

PREFACE
by Paul Lee

Ken Hancock is a bus supervisor in Derby, England. He reminds me of the British actor in *My Fair lady*, who sang: "Get Me to the Church on Time." A large, robust man with a music-hall sense of humour, he enjoys your double-take when you ask him if he is a professional herbalist, and he answers "bus supervisor."

The world's greatest living authority on Feverfew (*Tanacetum parthenium*(does it as a hobby, in his spare time. He set out to find an herbal, or natural, cure for his wife's migraines. The irony of it all was that she turned out to be allergic to the herb.

Feverfew cures headaches. I know from my own experience. I had heard about the British interest in the herb and the research that was reported in the literature, particularly *The Lancet*. Also, some was growing in my backyard, where my wife and I maintain an extensive garden of medicinal herbs.

My wife gets headaches rather frequently because she is light sensitive to the strong sub-tropical sun of Santa Cruz, California, where we live. I picked some Feverfew, made tea and her headache disappeared. Just like that! I figured there must be *something* to it.

Then I met Mr. Hancock, and he told me about the book he had written and his crusade to get the word out about Feverfew. His romance with a single herb reminded me about mine and herb thyme (*Thymus vulgaris*). It may not take one herb nut to recognize another, but I could tell that Ken Hancock knew what he was talking about from personal experience and the testimonials of thousands of people who have written to him abut Feverfew.

It is a fascinating and remarkable story he has to tell in order to introduce the American health consumer (and headache sufferer) to the merits of Feverfew. On this score, the testimonials reprinted in this book speak for themselves, even though scientific methodology regards them as mere anecdotes. No one knows if they are true or false. What is proof to Mr. Hancock is an unverified claim according to science.

The reader will approach this account with a growing sense of scepticism, beyond the issue of proof versus anecdote, when the discussion moves into psoriasis and arthritis. Mr. Hancock sees them as interrelated, along with the headaches and migraines, and speaks of them as the spectrum targeted by Feverfew.

Arthritis is a difficult disease state to approach because those engaged in its cure are so open to the suspicion of quackery. Herbs are already suspect, in principle, by health professionals, who regard them as archaic and obsolete. Many health workers have a functional disability in acknowledging the botanical basis of health care in medicinal herbs because they have received no training in the subject matter. Study of herbal medicine has been eliminated from the curriculum of health professional training in the United States.

This rejection defines the difference between folk medicine and industrial or, scientific, medicine. It is the difference between herbs and synthetic drugs.

Herbal health care, as folk medicine, has a sphere of validity all to itself. All traditional societies rely on it as the major form of health care. That means most of the people of the world. They cannot afford industrial medicine. They are dependent on the arts and crafts of the native healer who is usually an herbalist. The Spanish have a nice name for them—curanderos. For this reason, the World Health Organization has called for world-wide promotion and support of the herbalist in a move to provide health care for everyone in the world by the year 2000. This is only part of the reason why an "herb renaissance" is underway and why Americans are re-discovering the botanical basis of health care.

It is no surprise, then, that Ken Hancock went among the folk in his neighborhood, and especially English gardeners, to find out about Feverfew—which plants worked the best, in terms of varieties, and how to grow them. Think of it: the cure to many of your ills could be growing in your backyard. As Mr. Hancock mentions, you can grow a lifetime of Feverfew remedy with only a couple of plants.

It is a pleasure for me to introduce this book to an American readership. I am certain that the book will succeed in its mission, as the word is already out about Feverfew. The practical advice about dosage, about varieties, about methods of taking it, about the ramifications of Feverfew beyond its use as a headache cure, will fascinate the health consumer in this country who is looking for an herbal approach to health.

I share some of Mr. Hancock's views, such as "selective affinity," which sounds very much like Goethe, when I follow, in the tradition of Vitalism in botany. To account for this "selective affinity," I have postulated "an herb code in the immune memory of DNA," in an attempt to account for the relation between herbs and the human immune system. I would guess that much of Mr. Hancock's interest in the mode of action of Feverfew will come from the field of immunology, now that there are converging lines of international research on herbs that stimulate the immune system, our natural self-defense against illness and disease.

It will be an even greater pleasure if you respond to Mr. Hancock's invitation and tell him of your experiences with Feverfew. This will swell the tide of response to the benefits of the plant.

Eventually, science will provide the appropriate support for this folk remedy; this will be a task for pharmacognosy, a sub-division of pharmacology dealing specifically with the medicinal properties of herbs and their active constituents. Such research is already underway and is being reported in the scientific literature.

We have Mr. Hancock to thank for beating the drum for Feverfew. Through his dedication to this herb, together with assistance from his wife and his devoted friends, sufferers will now know of the herb and get the relief that has so long eluded them.

Thanksgiving, 1985

A NOTE ON THE BOTANY AND PHARMACOLOGY OF FEVERFEW

by Christopher Hobbs, Herbalist

Feverfew is a member of the second largest family among the flowering plants, the Daisy Family, or *Compositae*. Recently, some of the old family names have been changed to reflect a standardized ending of aceae, and consequently *Compositae* has become *Asteraceae* in some works. Many botanists still prefer the old name, and either one is correct. *Compositae* boasts some 18,000 species, or members, worldwide. This is second only to the Orchid Family, *Orchidaceae,* with over 20,000 members.

The family derives its name from the flowering part of its members, which is known as the inflorescence. In *Compositae*, the inflorescence, or flowering "head," is actually made up of several to hundreds of individual flowers. Think of a Sunflower head, where there are several hundred flowers, all insect pollinated. After pollination, the flowers fall off, revealing the many sunflower seeds.

The family of Feverfew includes the common garden plants, Black-eyed Susan, Cosmos and Marigold: the medicinal plants, Echinacea, Burdock and Calendula, and the edible Sunflower, Artichoke and Jerusalem artichoke.

More closely related to Feverfew are members of the genus Chrysanthemum: the common Chrysanthemum or "Mums" of florists' shops, *Chrysanthemum furtesens*; the common weed, Oxe-eye Daisy, *Chrysanthemum leucanthemum*, also an important Chinese herb; and the source of the insecticide pyrethrum, *Chrysanthemum cinerariaefolium*. In fact, the genus Chrysanthemum contains over 100 members, mostly from the Northern Hemisphere and the Old World. The name comes from the greek, *chrusos*, gold and *anthemon*, flower.

There are three or four varieties of Feverfew. L.H. Bailey, a renowned authority on horticultural matters, describes variety *crispum*, where the leaf edges are curled, and variety *aureum*, where the leaves are noticeably yellow. Besides this, there are several forms of the common wild variety, one with two or more rows of ray-flowers (the white pelaloid parts), one with no ray-flowers (where the heads have no white petals—only a yellow center) and the variety of Feverfew that has been subjected to extensive chemical and pharmacological testing having green leaves, with a touch of yellow and flowering heads with only *one* row of white ray flowers. This is the form that should be collected and used for any personal or commercial purposes.

The following is a description of the 'wild variety,' meaning that it grows wild and is not a nursery variety for ornament.

> Bushy perennial, 1–2 or 3 feet tall and much branched, especially above. Very leafy, with the nearly hairless leaves variably cut into sharp-pointed lobs (not linear segments, such as other Tanacetum species and Matricaria), and not usually over 3 inches long. The flowers are many in open terminal clusters and are about ¾" across. They have a single row of white rays (10–20), and a yellow center consisting of many disc flowers. The plant has a strong odor, especially when bruised.

Feverfew is a remarkable example of medical science learning from folk medicine. In England, where Feverfew is being used daily as a protective herb against migraine headaches and arthritis, thousands of people are finding relief where nothing from the pharmacists' shelves will work. It is estimated that one out of ten people suffer from some form of migraine, and millions more, from arthritis. Starting before 1978, people began trying Feverfew out of depression after suffering severe headaches, sometimes for twenty or thirty years.

As an important remedy, Feverfew was revered by the ancients. Dioscorides extolls its virtues for melancholy and congestion of the lungs. As a headache remedy it is not new, either. In 1633, the famous English herbalist, Gerard, speaks of it being effective for "them that are giddie in the head, and for the 'St. Anthony's fire,' to all inflammations and hot swellings." In 1772, John Hill, M.D. wrote in his *Family Herbal*: "In the worst headache this herb exceeds whatever else is known."

Meanwhile, it has taken seven years for Feverfew to become widely known in the United States, after many years of success among the people of England.

In October of 1978, the first of what was to be a series of articles on Feverfew over the next seven years appeared in *Lancet*, the prestigious British medical journal. At that time, not much was known of the chemistry, pharmacology or safety of long-term use. In 1980, the first scientific investigations were begun at the Miles Laboratory Ltd., led by H.O. Collier.

Because Feverfew has traditionally been used as a diaphoretic, to lower fevers, and because it had reputed success in cases of migraine headaches and arthritis, scientists hypothesized that the method of action on the body might be similar to aspirin, which is effective for similar ailments. Since it was known that aspirin, or acetylsalicylic acid, works by inhibiting the production of chemical agents in the body known as prostaglandins, it seemed likely that Feverfew was similar in its action.

Prostaglandins are chemical substances in the body present in minute amounts. There are many different kinds of prostaglandins, and they have many specific functions. They are well known to be local messengers, involved in the process of inflammation. Like aspirin and other salicylates, the active chemicals identified in Feverfew inhibit the production of prostaglandins, thus blocking or reducing inflammatory reactions in the body, determining how much blood is delivered to particular tissues. This is important, for it is the narrowing and widening of the blood vessels in the brain that has been linked with migraine headache; and the inflammatory process itself that causes the pain, swelling and even disfiguration of joints and other tissues in arthritis. Feverfew has been shown to help reduce pain in cases of arthritis.

The narrowing of the blood vessels reduces the blood supply to parts of the brain, such as the visual center, causing symptoms such as blurred vision. Expansion, or dilation of the vessels, can produce the feeling of fullness or pressure and pounding that most headache sufferers experience.

An interesting note is that the main active chemical in Feverfew, which has been named parthenolide, inhibits not only prostaglandins, but also the recently discovered leukotrienes, which are slow-reacting substances that stimulate allergic reactions. These facts are thought by some scientists to explain the diverse range of beneficial activities attributed to Feverfew.

Besides these, Feverfew herb has also been demonstrated to inhibit other substances, called amines, specifically, serotonin, noradrenalin and histamine. These substances are known to increase in the brain during the early phase of migraine attack. Incidentally, certain foods, known as "trigger" foods, contain similar amines and are known to initiate a migraine episode. These foods include coffee, chocolate and some fried foods.

Parthenolide is not stable when subjected to high heat. This means that the best preparations of Feverfew are ones that are produced with as little heat as possible. The best choice is freeze-drying. Freeze-dried herb was used successfully in a double-blind trial with migraine sufferers, reducing headaches and other unpleasant symptoms of migraine as effectively as the fresh leaves, the most common way of taking Feverfew. Freeze-dried capsules or tablets would have the additional advantages of ease of taking the herb and having a portable supply of the herb to take on trips. Many migraine sufferers have been limited in traveling because of the fear of being away from a fresh supply of Feverfew. Carefully dried herb has been shown to be effective, but many may not be as good. Heating the herb in the preparation of teas, or improper drying, could inactivate the beneficial properties.

Feverfew had an additional advantage as a treatment for migraine and arthritis. Unlike aspirin, which is the most common drug used in these ailments, Feverfew has few or no demonstrable side-effects. Aspirin can cause bleeding in the stomach and is not indicated for anyone with ulcers or internal hemorrhage. Feverfew has shown no severe side-effects over the 6-year period that long-term users have been checked for blood pressure, liver function and other important tests. The only noticeable undesirable effects have been mouth and throat irritation in allergic reactions.

THE FEVERFEW STORY

In the Beginning, "FEVERFEW"

Alternative medicine is a 20th century term which refers to herbal or homeopathic medicine, acupuncture, osteopathy, etc., despite the fact that such treatments have been available for thousands of years, with the exception of homeopathy. Orthodox or synthetic medicine, having been with us for decades only, should really bear the title alternative medicine. But since the advent of World War II, based on the undeniable impact of penicillin, alternative—or folk medicine as I prefer to call it—has been pushed firmly into the background. Due to the considerable impact now being made by certain herbs, a renaissance of folk medicine is imminent, synthetic medicine having failed to compete successfully in the specific area of involvement of these herbs.

This book is directed specifically at disclosing the curative powers of one variety of herb, *Tanacetum parthenium*. The herb is not new to herbal medicine, nor is this variety of hybrid developed for the treatment of specific ailments. It is, however, a *wild* variety of Feverfew. Possible interbreeding has caused considerable variation in the medicinal qualities of this type of Feverfew by comparison with other types. The herb has been in medicinal use for millennia. It was very popular with the medieval herbal physicians of England, who spoke very highly of it.

Unfortunately, there has been little of consequence written in general terms about the efficacy of Feverfew since the 17th century. There have been a number of scientific papers, but they have had little impact on the layperson. Until comparatively recently the medical establishment has fought fiercely to prevent folk medicine from becoming acceptable treatment again.

It is entirely possible that interest in this field has been sparked off anew in areas where synthetic medicine has not only failed to provide an answer, but in the course of trials has provided frightful side-effects. This, in turn, has given people a deep-seated fear of synthetic medicine, to the extent that many have chosen to suffer rather than accept the attendant risks. A great deal of publicity has been given in recent years to the side-effects of certain synthetic drugs, and to the supposedly foolproof tests that gain them admission to the drug register. This fear of synthetics is very real:

> *'My wife and I have for some time suffered pain and swelling from arthritis, and were very reluctant to take pain-*

killing drugs since the very bad experience of a friend who is now in a wheelchair.' Testimonial 3.

'I was taking 6 aspirins daily and capsules from my doctor. The pain was unbearable, but the side-effects were so severe that I could only take the capsules two days at a time.' Testimonial 6.

'I did not wish to try strong drugs, with side-effects probably worse than my symptoms.' Testimonial 45.

These are typical of many letters received during the course of my research. I have sympathy for medical professionals generally, for they are undoubtedly in a cleft stick; they know better than anyone that they have nothing more than painkillers to offer in all too many cases.

Unfortunately, the attitude of "orthodoxy" is inconsistent in its approach to folk medicine. On the one hand, we have practitioners prepared to keep an open mind, who are aware that the laboratories can provide no alternative and, subject to obvious safeguards, are prepared to revert to herbal medicine where necessary. This is not confined solely to general practitioners, nor to herbs, for certain hospitals are currently testing the effectiveness of leeches in post-surgical situations. I well remember an old Tamil bearer picking leeches off my body after my return from duty in the Malayan jungle. He put them into a jam jar, and I asked why he wanted them; his reply was "Very good price in town, sahib, only take bad blood." At that time I wasn't particularly bothered why he wanted them, but his reply is firmly registered in my memory 29 years later.

On the other hand there are the die-hards who will admit to no good whatsoever in connection with folk medicine, dismissing it as ignorant, superstitious nonsense. They will have nothing to do with it, their only guide to treatment being the drug laboratory handbook. The vast majority of herbal treatments are perfectly safe even in unpracticed hands; just a little commonsense is required. Possible side-effects have been recorded throughout centuries of use, but some doctors prefer to continue the usage of drugs known to have violent or at the very least distressing side-effects, without giving relief.

This is not intended to imply that Feverfew does not have its problems, but to date I have not been able to discover anything more serious than allergic reaction, the symptoms of which are temporary. I am in touch with various research teams in the U.K. and abroad, and so far they have not discovered anything untoward. Quite the contrary, Feverfew is not on the official list of drugs requiring further investigation by virtue of having suspected toxicity problems. Allergic reaction affects approximately 7% of leaftakers and 2% of users of manufactured products.

Fresh leaf is obviously the most direct form of treatment and the cheapest, because two or three plants will provide a supply for an individual lifetime. It is unfortunate that this form also has the highest incidence of allergic reaction, is difficult to assess relative to accurate dosage, and is not particularly convenient. Nevertheless, it has a great following. Manufacturers of herbal products, aware of these problems, make dried Feverfew into tablets or capsules, and homeopathic essences from fresh leaf.

During a visit to a laboratory two years ago, after giving an opinion on the type and quality of Feverfew being used, I was given the freedom of the laboratory, and I was agreeably surprised to discover the degree of expertise and care that was evident. Naturally, it is necessary to ensure that the variety of herb is correct, but other safeguards were stringently applied. Optimum harvesting time is important with Feverfew; freedom from foreign inclusions, or containmants such as herbicides or pesticides and lead from petrol fumes, is an additional safeguard in all cases.

Supplies of herb brought in from abroad have been suspect for some time, and it is not always possible or advisable to rely on certificates of authenticity. Sophisticated technology makes possible discrimination between milled Feverfew and Camomile, for example. In addition this same technology has revealed that potentially harmful plants have not been removed prior to the drying and milling processes in some cases. For this reason, the reputable laboratories either grow the herb themselves or obtain it by contract from reputable growers. A process now available in the United States guarantees that *all* foreign inclusions, including minute insects and dust, will be removed during the drying process.

Air-dried Feverfew is proving to be as effective as fresh leaf without causing as many allergy problems. The process in the United States also promises to give exceptional results, and I am eager to test the level of activity and rate of allergic incidence against that of current products.

A barrier to world-wide sales thus far has been the insistence of many manufacturers in the U.K. on using animal-based fillers, e.g., bone phosphate. This does not affect the performance of the herb, but it does restrict sales because some religions forbid such practices, and vegetarians will not take them. This practice is now under review, and the U.K.

should soon fall into line with those countries where mineral filler is considered normal practice. Capsules do not cause problems in this respect, but they are normally more expensive.

Varieties of Feverfew

In the U.K., there are four main varieties of Feverfew; regional or soil variations have an effect on leaf identification but not on the flower. These variations have little effect on the medicinal qualities of Feverfew, but I feel that interbreeding of the wild variety has had a considerable effect on its medicinal qualities, for it stands head and shoulders above the others.

Golden Feverfew is the best known variety of the cultivated type, but it has little to commend it as a medicinal plant in comparison with the wild variety. It will give relief from migraine, but it will not touch arthritis or psoriasis, and in general it is slow and unreliable.

This variety has given me many problems in the past because people have used it without correctly identifying it, and having received no benefit they write to tell me that Feverfew does not work. I have always specified *Tanacetum parthenium* since my initial research was concluded, over seven years ago.

> *'I feel that I must write and tell you that since I started taking the correct Feverfew the pain in my arms and back has gone completely.' Testimonial 174.*

> *'I'm so very glad that I sent for your broadsheet and especially so since I had been taking Golden Feverfew without result for 6 months.' Testimonial 268.*

Tanacetum parthenium is the name most preferred by experts in connection with Wild Feverfew, but specialists have informed me that it is also known as *Chrysanthemum parthenium*, and *Matricaria parthenium*. This will be the only reference to these alternative names in this book, for they have caused much confusion over the years. I would much prefer that as far as the medicinal application is concerned, it should be known as either *Tanacetum parthenium* or Wild Feverfew.

Local knowledge

A knowledge of the medicinal qualities of Feverfew is widespread throughout the U.K. Many will doubt that this is true judging by the number of enquiries I have received requesting information: in excess of 40,000 in nine years, the bulk of them in 1984. The herb is well known however, but the knowledge is confined to certain communities or isolated pockets. Only occasionally does someone put pen to paper and pass the knowledge on, which is a great pity, for the herb has so much to offer and so little vice.

> *'I was recommended to take Feverfew by an old coal miner, who said that his colleagues often ate it to relieve them of headaches by being underground in poor conditions of ventilation.' Testimonial 246.*

> *'I am one of the many people who have found relief from Feverfew since your letters were published last year.' Testimonial 5.*

Why research Feverfew?

A point of interest in many letters has been the reason for my dedication to Feverfew in particular, whilst apparently ignoring other herbal treatments. It is a factor that for many years before I grew attached to this herb, I had been subjected from time to time to country remedies, basically for the relief of congestion, but it was not until 1976 that I had reason to develop a major interest.

In that year a friend of my wife gave her a magazine clipping that mentioned Feverfew as a possible cure for migraine. It did not come from a scientific magazine; rather, it was a general publication that just happened to have an interest in passing on a bit of country lore. Unfortunately, it was not specific relative to the type of Feverfew or dosage to be taken.

The friend knew that for many years my wife had been sadly afflicted with migraine, and nothing available in orthodox or synthetic medicine had helped. The migraines came and went with monotonous regularity, but the crippling pain during an attack was not the only associated problem: the anticipation of pain on a regular timetable was an aggravating influence for days prior to the actual attack, and the aftermath was prolonged. In effect, my wife was free from pain, or the effects of pain, for few consecutive days.

I do not need to tell anyone closely related to a migraine sufferer of the effect of migraine on family life, but a considerable number of testimonials sent to me by former sufferers stress this point. So many times parents have said that they wish that they had heard of Feverfew earlier in life, because they would have been able to enjoy the company of their children in their formative years, instead of shutting themselves away in a darkened room most of the time.

Although the major concern in the case of my wife was migraine, psoriasis was a close second. Much of the unsightly scale caused by this disease was clearly evident in normal dress. Beach clothes or swimsuits were definitely out. There was no pain factor to consider, but as a stress problem, it was a continuous aggravation to the migraine problem. Once again, she had taken advantage of available treatment, to no avail. In some areas of the body, the effects were seasonal, but the overall effect was permanent. It is interesting to recall that at the age of 15, when we first met, the twin problems of psoriasis and migraine were both present and clearly evident. At the time I had no definite interest in herbal medicine and certainly no concept that the problems might be related by common cause.

We were well into married life before we entered into detailed discussion regarding the psoriasis, and my wife freely admitted to an inferiority complex because of it. The ailment had begun to manifest itself shortly after an operation for an eye defect at the age of 7 years. Virtually from the onset of the problem, doctors and clinics had offered lotions and potions for external treatment, but they admitted that no permanent cure, or even the cause, was known. They did say that it was believed to be the result of excess acid in the blood.

Later in life, my wife began to exhibit symptoms of arthritis in her knees and fingers, but this was still pre-Feverfew, and I did not appreciate the implications of the onset of this ailment. She did inform me at this time that a clinic in Birmingham, England, had been quite successful in clearing psoriasis during one set of clinical trials, but that the result of the treatment had been to cause arthritis to appear and become dominant. This simple statement was of only passing interest at the time, for I had not yet begun to appreciate the tripartite agreement between the three ailments mentioned thus far, either by cause or incidence.

As Feverfew has not helped my wife, she could easily be forgiven for washing her hands of the entire project, but this has not been the case. She has witnessed the effects of the herb, and she naturally has access to the visitors who call to tell us of their success with the herb. Within one period of three days whilst I was at work, she personally answered the door to two professional pianists who had been able to resume playing due to the herb.

Better than anyone else I know, she can isolate the most active of the range of Feverfew varieties in our garden. She does this by taste alone, and throughout the growing season she pronounces on relative strengths. As far as level of activity is concerned she might run a close second to a chromatograph scan.

In doing this evaluation, which is quite voluntary, she invariably ends up with a sore mouth for a few days, but she will not desist. I have watched her wade into Feverfew plants in civic gardens on the continent of Europe to test the strength of Feverfew plants she has spotted. On one occasion the variety was so powerful that I wrote to the Mayor of the town in order to contact the horticultural head to obtain seeds. These worthies were most helpful, and the seeds are growing merrily.

I live in hope that one day I shall be able to offer my wife a viable alternative to Feverfew, or that some change in body chemistry will enable her to take the herb; for the present she remains one of the few who are allergic to it.

Initial research

Following the acquisition of the magazine clipping, I set off in high hopes of purchasing Feverfew, but to my dismay I could not find a single commercial product. A few herbalists had heard of it, but none sold it. Even large herbal houses told me that it did not appear in their lists of medicinal herbs. At this stage, I was obligated to turn to the medieval literature of England, and there in the works attributed to Culpeper and Gerard I found it. They were particularly fond of the herb, and mention it amongst other ailments as being efficacious in the case of "the worst headache known," an obvious reference to migraine.

Since I am not a keen gardener and can identify little more than Daffodils or Tulips, I set off down the road to a country manor house not far from my home. There in the herb garden, with the kind and willing assistance of a gardener, Jeff, by name, I found one variety of the herb. Jeff told me that he had heard that the herb might be useful for migraine sufferers. He then offered a plant and told me that another country house approximately 25 miles away grew another variety.

And so this was the pattern established from then on. I was passed from hand to hand, from Mr. X to Mrs. Y who might know more. Although I appreciated the assistance of these kindly people, I did not realize at the time how deeply indebted I would become later in my research. They gave of their time and innumerable cups of tea quite freely, whilst relating invaluable personal experiences. In the beginning I was concerned only with the effect of the herb relative to migraine, but it very soon became obvious that I could no longer consider this ailment in isolation, at least as far as one variety of the herb was concerned; this was Wild Feverfew.

During my conversations with these friendly people arthritis was mentioned, and I began to ask questions instead of merely listening. It was not my intention to put words into their mouths, but as with my wife it may have been that only one ailment was considered, with secondary benefit being taken for granted.

As a result, at the end of 18 months of research I gained reasonably comprehensive knowledge of the medicinal qualities of Feverfew in its various forms. It would have been very easy to continue with the research for its own sake, but the primary reason for the work was the problem experienced by my wife, and my plants had grown to maturity; I was satisfied that she would not come to harm by using the herb. So my wife took her Feverfew leaves and tragedy struck. I was naturally aware of the allergic reaction experienced by some people, but as with accidents I considered that it could only happen to other people. This time I was unlucky. My wife revealed the classic symptoms of allergic reaction. She waited for a week and tried again, in case the reaction had been caused by something else, but the result was the same.

To say that I was dismayed is to understate the case; I was heartbroken. I knew that the answer was there in Feverfew, but she could not use it. Being a creature of impulse I immediately consigned my notes to the care and consideration of the garden incinerator. Thank goodness the incinerator could not erase my memory, for only a short while later a colleague, who was severely afflicted with arthritis, asked if I would give him a plant and the information for its use.

He began treatment with the knowledge and assistance of his doctor, and seven days from commencement he told me that his pain was greatly reduced. I smiled and said that he should tell me after a month, but he was soon back, reporting that his soreness, swelling and inflammation were also reduced, and that his mobility was increasing. I knew through my research that this was a reasonably average pattern, but I was very concerned at the possibility of placebo action. Now I have so much proof of the efficacy of the herb, and I have lost count of the times health food shopkeepers have told me of visits by doctors to purchase tablets for their own use.

My colleague continued treatment, and benefit was progressive as far as arthritis and sleeping problems were concerned. He had taken many synthetic drugs, but with the co-operation of his doctor these were reduced to an absolute minimum, and he is now retired in excellent health. I see him from time to time, and quite apart from other activities he is still fully engrossed with Feverfew, his greenhouse madly growing plants for other sufferers.

Progress was slow after the initial case, simply because I did not immediately set out my stall to tell all, but the ball began rolling because of this one individual. Today I receive letters from the far corners of the earth, and correspondence takes up all my spare time. I hope that this book will save time in providing answers to questions, leaving me free to pursue other facets of Feverfew.

In the Beginning, "Feverfew"

The principle of homeostasis

'I had also suffered severe migraine since my second child was born. Testimonial 192.

'For many years since the birth of our son many years ago, she has suffered from continual cracking and splitting of the finger nail. On all her fingers the nail split almost down to the quick.' Testimonial 237.

'Being a sufferer of lower back pain and for some years in the neck and shoulders as the result of a motor accident, I purchased a box of tablets. After taking one a day for about 3 weeks I have received much relief. The back pain vanished almost immediately.' Testimonial 234.

These letters are typical of many; individuals can recall an incident that affected them deeply shortly before the onset of the ailments. I say ailments, although it is possible that only one ailment revealed itself initially, to be followed by one or other related ailment at a later date. Severe pain during childbirth, the death of a family member or close friend, an accident or operation are all mentioned as traumatic experiences known to have occurred at the critical time.

I have heard it said many times that arthritis followed an accident, but it is perfectly clear that what is uppermost in the minds of these people is the physical impact involved. The impression given is that of the effect of a hammer hitting an egg. The sheer percussion effect is the cause of the onset of arthritis, but while I am not prepared to argue the case of the egg, I feel that the physical impact in the case of bodily injury is secondary to the mental impact. Even though bones are broken or severely bruised, this does not explain why migraine and psoriasis may arise as a result of the same trauma. The effect of trauma is to cause glandular imbalance, which in turn manifests itself in the form of arthritis, psoriasis or migraine in so many cases.

At one stage in my research I suggested to a learned gentleman that, in view of the minute quantity of Feverfew ingested compared with the magnificent, often virtually immediate beneficial results, the majority of the work must be performed by the body's own self-repair mechanism. It is the ability of herbs to drive directly at a point of selective affinity that makes them so effective, and by curing an imbalance in a particular area they may be responsible for relief in a number of seemingly unrelated illnesses.

On the surface arthritis, migraine, and psoriasis are seemingly unrelated, but they do share the common factor of stress as a continuing state, and as often as not a common factor—the trauma—occurring shortly before the onset of the problems. We can look at the factor of stress in two ways, however: as a contributory cause to the onset of the ailment, or as a consequence of the ailment. The first is hypothetical to a point, but the second must be accepted as a fact, since nobody will attempt to deny the effect of pain and distress caused by the three ailments mentioned.

Why should a traumatic situation be responsible for a purely physical ailment? The brain is an extremely efficient instrument, but like any other computer it requires data input to cope with a given situation. Some of this knowledge is hereditary. Consider the plight of the North American Indian as the pioneers trekked Westward. Unlike the pioneers, the Indian had no data bank of knowledge concerning chickenpox, and the necessary antibodies were not forthcoming. The body's defense system could not even begin to organize a defense, and the Indians were decimated. Today, because of hereditary knowledge, the information is available, because of exposure, and the Indian suffers little more than anyone else. This has been repeated many times in many centuries throughout the world, as the "civilized" world spread its "benefits" during conquering forays.

Because the principle of homeostasis applies, the brain can cope once information is input; specific antibodies can be produced to cope with specific situations. But are we entitled to believe that the brain responds to trauma automatically, that the information is already available? I think not because trauma is entirely personal, and we cannot expect the brain to deal with it as with chickenpox. We should not expect evolution to have provided information to deal with this problem, and we certainly must not take for granted hereditary protection against its effects.

If we assume that the brain has the necessary data to permit remedial action to be taken, we must also assume that if the remedial action is not forthcoming, there is a breakdown in communication somewhere down the line. Work Centre 1 has not received instructions, a fuse has blown somewhere, and the chemical messengers are not sent out to the organs that should make a contribution. The breakdown may be within Work Centre 1, so that even if the relevant work permits have been issued there is no chance of the work being done.

Wherever the breakdown occurs it is the common point of affinity through which Feverfew works; this is the point in the physiological system that is the whole *raison d'etre* of Feverfew.

I believe that once Feverfew has reached this point, communications begin to flow again, and the principle of feedback as defined in homeostasis begins to take over. This refers to a system whereby information fed into the brain will have an effect on the concentration of substances in the blood amongst other things. We are told that certain substances in the blood if produced in excess will cause soreness, inflammation and swelling; we are also told that in a dangerous situation the adrenalin flows, and this is true of any stressful situation. But what if the adrenalin does not flow simply because nobody has been able to reach the adrenal gland, to give it a bit of overtime?

Accepting that in general the bloodstream is the carrier of corrective substances to all parts of the body and that the final link in the chain of events that Feverfew provokes is the change in the white cell blood groups, we still have not established why the correction was not put in hand automatically. We are in effect trying to discover the common point of affinity with the ailments.

Feverfew does not cause similar beneficial effects in all cases within a set time scale. The response of biological systems is usually variable relative to information entered, and so there may be as many responses as there are people on this planet. When one takes into account other potential variables such as residual drugs that are not part of the physiological system, the number of possible combinations is multiplied enormously.

Early steps in synthetics

Claims have been made that by means of molecular restructuring anything may be duplicated artificially, but if this is so why have we not yet got artificial Feverfew? I have no doubt that attempts have been going on long enough, but we are still waiting. The fact is that the herb consistently defies a breakdown of the full implication of its constituent parts, yet claims have been made that it is now possible to extract those parts that make it effective. Does a body live without a soul, and is not the balance of Feverfew its very soul?

My opinion is that we should not expect early synthesization of Feverfew, for although it may well be possible to extract some of its constituent parts, it is not yet possible to duplicate the soul of Feverfew, and without this soul, this natural balance, I believe the herb could be as lethal as certain synthetic drugs. I would even argue against the removal of that isolate of Feverfew that causes allergic reaction, because I believe it is there for a purpose.

It was not until well into the 20th century that synthetic drugs began to play a major role in medicine, but although it was World War II that gave the necessary stimulus for research into the benefits of penicillin, the process of synthesization was already established. Paul Ehrlich discovered that certain tissues have a selective affinity for certain chemicals; the development of arsphenamine was a major step, and although it was an early advance into synthetic medicine, I believe it is at this stage that we see the birth of the modern drug industry. Feverfew takes a step backward with the remainder of the medicinal herbs.

Because of the principle of selective affinity, however, we can begin to understand how Feverfew may succeed where modern drugs fail. In a way, I am answering a question I put to you earlier, regarding the principle by which synthetic drugs perform their function. It is becoming clear that synthetics must have a specific aiming point; if they are not told where to go they cannot do their job. So if nobody knows where to send them there is little point in introducing them to the system.

The principle of selective affinity is the basis of herbal treatment, for each herb knows precisely where to go and what to do when it gets there. For this reason, it is not necessary to consume mountains of Feverfew—just enough to get the job done, and a little to keep the wheels turning, in some cases, but not in all. One might be entitled to believe that having reached this stage in herbal technology, a little effort might have been directed towards the reinstatement of folk medicine, but the attitude appears to be, why grow it if you can make it? An admirable sentiment if you can make it, but we are still awaiting a synthetic cure for arthritis, migraine, psoriasis and stress, while Feverfew sits quietly in the background, helping the few instead of the multitude.

As if arsphenamine was not enough, the 1930s saw the development of the sulphonamide group of drugs directed specifically at infections of the bloodstream. As this group evolved, variations on the theme became numerous, and as with any group of synthetics thousands of experiments were required to produce very few acceptable drugs. Folk medicine took another step backwards into relative obscurity.

An experiment that interests me greatly is that of Paul Hench and his group in Minnesota. The experiment was undertaken more in the interests of synthetic medicine, but it does have a very important bearing on my theory regarding the prime function of Feverfew. Hench's group discovered that a substance which they called compound E could be isolated from the cortex of the adrenal glands. We know it as cortisone. Hench believed that it would provide a cure for rheumatoid arthritis. This was not to be, unfortunately, despite the undoubted anti-inflammatory properties of the substance.

Despite the apparent failure of the overall conception, the discovery of a method which permitted the identification and isolation of compound E was a great step forward, but only part of the answer. It falls into the same category as the behaviour of certain white cell groups as they come within the influence of Feverfew; it is an important factor but not the complete answer. These individual discoveries are vital steps along the path toward a full realization of the value of Feverfew. The scientific tests now being undertaken are more akin to my own research in many ways, because there is far more emphasis on the effects of the herb, instead of on particular isolates. By studying effects it is more likely that the selective point of affinity will be isolated. This is essential if we are to learn more about the herb.

According to the principle of enzymatic homeostatis, we are given to understand that the adverse results of deficient enzymatic activity may lead to a breakdown in communications. This breakdown may affect the function of operator genes to the extent that they are not prompted or allowed to complete their task of instigating activity in structural genes. I put to you the possibility that this deficiency may be likened to the breakdown of a neural fuse, or at the very least is complementary to it.

Hench would undoubtedly have been familiar with the example of enzymatic deficiency known as adrenogenital syndrome, which is caused by the lack of an enzyme that has a place in the synthesis of cortisone, a deficiency that leads to a failure of proper control of adrenal activity. Is the missing enzyme incorporated into Feverfew?

The true function of Feverfew

We have now arrived at the stage where we may analyze the way in which Feverfew fulfills its function. Those people who advocate individual facets of the herb's behaviour have failed to grasp the entire picture. There is very little point in looking at only a part of the whole, because it can be misleading and time-consuming.

The work of the Minnesota group is an important part, but if Paul Hench had been working along the lines suggested by Feverfew his next step would have been an investigation either into another facet of the herb's involvement chemically, or an attempt to relate other ailments to the same area. Consider the effect if another team had been working alongside on the function of Feverfew. It would have been a splendid opportunity to examine the herb, and to assess whether or not the herb did affect the synthesis of compound E; would he have found the missing enzyme in Feverfew?

It is even possible that had he known about the effect of Feverfew as revealed in the testimonials sent to me, he may have cracked the problem wide open. The regulatory aspect of Feverfew involvement is all-important in the function of the herb. Its effect on glandular activity, with or without the cooperation of the brain, is of primary importance. It may be that certain remedial work has to be undertaken before the brain can commence its own duties, and if a neural fuse has blown this would most certainly be the case.

I do believe that the brain is ultimately responsible for controlling the complex mixture of substances stimulated by Feverfew, and obviously for passing these substances to the affected areas. Its duties would probably also include the integration of the substances as the relevant stimuli reach affected glands.

Like any other regulator, Feverfew will be responsible for increased or reduced flow. In the case of psoriasis if there is an excess of acid in the blood we have two alternatives to consider. Either the herb neutralizes the acid to an acceptable level, but this would require considerable ingestion, or it regulates the output of acid by exercising its influences on the unbalanced gland responsible for the over-production.

It can be seen that the herb exerts considerable influence on soreness, swelling and inflammation. We have further alternatives to consider. The first is that Feverfew reduces the output of inflammatory substances, and the second is that it controls the effect of these substances by increasing the output of compound E. I believe the first to be the case, for simply to cover the effects of an imbalance is not the function of herbs. Feverfew is quite capable of two-way regulation, but the increased capability is more complex than the reduction capability. It would appear that the herb is quite happy to reduce the levels of unwanted or unnecessary substances, but it increases the output of desirable substances in closely controlled combination.

The results of my research have shown a positive link between arthritis, migraine, psoriasais and stress. I contend that these ailments share a common cause. It may well be in the end that I shall be proved wrong, and that Feverfew merely shares a common point of selective affinity with the other ailments. By exercising its regulatory function in common ground, Feverfew is efficacious in multi-ailment relief. Whatever the result, I shall be satisfied that relief will be found for sufferers.

Why do I stress this common point of selective affinity? At present we have various organizations delving into research to individual ailments, but I know of none dedicated to research into common ground. I sincerely hope that my research will instigate a new approach, even of minor dimensions. I have been asked for information from time to time, by various research facilities, but each asks for a particular facet, none for the whole, and research patterns remain as divergent as ever. I would like to see more cooperation between these individual teams, so that the end product could be expected sooner rather than later, for the benefit of all concerned. Let us take a step backwards and take the wider view. The common ground is there to be found.

Beneficial effects of Feverfew

It should have become apparent by now that my approach to Feverfew is totally different from that of most researchers. Once I was convinced that Feverfew was safe I set out to discover what it could do, not why it did it—although as you have already seen, I am now as concerned with function as with effect.

Most of the people I spoke to in the early days were country folk, born and bred; they knew the difference between safe herbs and dangerous ones, so they did not mind at all when I stressed safety. They would probably have been surprised if I hadn't. I mention this at this stage in case you should think that in my search for proof of benefit, I have avoided the possibility of adverse reaction. The benefits detailed in the following pages are divided into two categories.

Group 1 lists ailments for which I have substantial proof of Feverfew's benefits in the form of testimonials gathered over the years. At the back of the book you will find a selection of these testimonials—in edited form because most are too long to include in full—taken from those that arrived during the 6 months preceding the writing of this book. In this group you will find arthritis, migraine, psoriasis, and stress.

Group 2 is a miscellaneous group for which proof of Feverfew's effects exists but not in sufficient quantity to satisfy requirements for inclusion in Group 1.

GROUP 1

Arthritis

I confine myself to those types of arthritis mentioned in testimonials. There may well be more, but for the time being we shall consider osteo-arthritis, rheumatoid arthritis and ankylosing spondilitus. These three figure in claims of relief, but the first two in far greater numbers than the third.

I have seen many distressing sights during my research. Some of them have brought me to the verge of tears, not only because of the severe effects of arthritis on the human frame, but because of the patience and fortitude displayed by so many of the people affected. As if the pain and disability were not enough, many of them have told me that they feel totally rejected by society because of it. Whether they are so rejected I am not prepared to discuss, but my impression is that the feeling might not be so acute if it did not appear to begin with the doctor. "It is incurable and you will just have to learn to live with it." This sentence appears in so many letters, and while I could agree that it might simply be misquoted in a few cases, this cannot be true of all. One might believe that it is included in the medical textbook, but I know that the majority of doctors are not hard, unfeeling people. I feel that embarrassment at not being able to offer either a cure or hope of a cure may cause them to be a little gruff, but not unfeeling.

My own panel of doctors are lovely people, even though they are not afraid to say that they consider me to be a nut-case about herbs, but I have never had the opportunity to see how they cope with the problem. Because they so often adopt the self-defensive attitude mentioned, I ask any doctor who reads this book to accept the fact that this feeling of rejection is a major problem with many patients and to remember that the bedside manner is important.

> *'The doctor diagnosed my illness as a type of arthritis, inflammation of the tendons. . . . One looks around at friends and neighbours, aware how easily others' illness becomes boring.*
> *Feverfew, Ken Hancock, Kathy and Jack Turner = a hand stretched out to help, psychologically invaluable initially. . . . It seems new sufferers and those with no one to talk to need desperately someone to talk to who understands the shock of learning they are incurable. How to accept the rejection of one's own doctor, with nothing to offer except painkillers, when coming apart at the seams; they need strong support to help them rebuild morale fibre and readjust a way of living. . . . but it's coming and I'm fighting back now. Ken Hancock, Kathy and Jack Turner and Feverfew have provided invaluable first aid!'* Testimonial 262.

This letter puts into a nutshell the feelings of most people when faced with the prospect of progressive deterioration; it is not as if the lady asked for much—only treatment that could affect a fair proportion of the world's population. With the number of modern drugs available, she probably felt that her request was reasonable. How can we even begin to assess our personal reaction to the trauma this lady experienced, unless we have already been subjected to severe traumatic situations? It is not necessary to have undergone the same experience, to understand that to the person concerned it is of earth-shaking consequence. It may be that the lady herself had not come across a similar situation involving another person, for these sufferers do tend to isolate themselves for reasons already mentioned, and her own case would be the worse for this lack of experience. We can all help somebody else if we really want to, but some people in need are not too easy to find, strange as it may seem, especially when they deliberately hide themselves away.

The lady who wrote the above letter is lively, intelligent and imaginative, basically very strong mentally. She is an authoress, and her reaction was all the more powerful because of her imagination. Let me give you two more examples of reaction to a similar problem.

> *'For the past 2 years the use of my legs became a torture, so bad in fact that only rare days during the past year I've been able to walk. I'd shuffle, have to stop, pain tearing at me, feeling like a fool standing there unable to move, tears streaming down my face. Then I read a tiny bit of information about you. I did not believe it BUT I was so depressed and desperate I'd try anything, because believe me if I was to wind up in a wheelchair a large dose of sleeping tablets would be my only way out. When I give you my background you will understand that I'm no coward.' Testimonial 1.*

The lady did go on to tell me her background in a letter eight pages long. Those portions included in this book have been carefully edited to avoid chance of recognition, for she has been much in the public eye. My reward? The satisfaction of having helped her and a beautiful autographed photograph, which I can't put on the wall because of visitors. Jack Turner cried when I showed him my photograph, so I had to write and ask for one for him as well.

The next letter has been included not only because of the degree of distress it reveals but also because it answers so many potential questions relevant to age, degree of distress and the period over which this distress has been present.

> *'I've had arthritis first in the coccyx of the spine in 1940; 4 doctors gave me the news that nothing could be done . . . then I had what doctors called a frozen left shoulder in 1964, suffered intense pain, eventually told osteoarthritis and had a plastic shoulder in 1973, told then it was in my spine as well, have been trying every tablet on and off since. . . . I*

told the surgeon at xxxxxx Hospital that had it not been for my darling dog I would have ended my life. . . . I am 82 but I still believe in miracles.' Testimonial 208.

There is much more to this letter. You can read at the back of the book what Feverfew did for this lady. She is not the oldest person to have received benefit, but consider what she endured. The letter was sent to me in November 1984, almost 45 years after the onset of the problem.

You will find many testimonials referring both osteo and rheumatoid arthritis, but the effect of spondylitus is not so well corroborated, possibly because it is not as common as the other two.

'I have suffered with ankylosing spondylitis for 3 years (since 18), and I started to take Feverfew 2 months ago after having to take steroids to get me through my wedding day. It is great to find something that gives the relief without the side effects.'
Testimonial 96

On a less happy note, I spoke to a man last week who had taken Feverfew for one month who claimed that he had received no benefit. He has had his health problem for years, he is saturated with drugs, but he expected overnight relief. You can imagine my reply to him, and since he is male he was not accorded the same respect that I accord to the fairer sex of whatever age. He has now embarked on a fair trial.

Does Feverfew cure or merely relieve? Some technical people have said that it merely fulfills the function of "medieval aspirin" but if this were its only function then it is the longest lasting painkiller I know. I do know that the first person to try it in my personal experience does still top-up (sporadic ingestion to maintain relief) occasionally during the year, and I know that others wait until they get the odd ache before topping-up, often at intervals of 8 or 9 months. If I am right in my basic hypotheses, when the problem recurs, it is not the old pain back but a new series.

How effective is the relief?

An elderly woman came to see me shortly before Christmas 1983. Her problem was obvious: clenched useless fists. I was distressed when she told me that her fingernails had dropped off following treatment with a certain drug. It served me right for jumping to conclusions; the problem was not so much that her hands were crippled. The patience of this old lady was amazing. She wanted no recriminations for those who had used her as a human guinea pig; her hope was simply that one day she might obtain relief. But in the meantime she would press on regardless; and press on she did until she received a letter from her daughter in Canada.

It was an invitation to spend Christmas and New Year's in Canada. When the daughter emigrated, the mother's arthritis had not been at such an advanced stage, and the mother's only thought was the effect that her hands might have on her daughter and family. She came to see me because somebody had told her that Feverfew might help and she wanted to know more about it. The next communication I had from her was a post card from Canada in which she told me how much she had enjoyed her meal on the plane, knife, fork and all, and her turkey dinner at Christmas with her family. I see her occasionally as I go about my daily duties in the centre of Derby. She gives me a lovely smile, waggles her fingers and moves on; she knows it's enough.

On odd occasions when sceptics expressed doubt, I provide a box of testimonials, a comfortable chair and tell them to get reading. One couple sat through a night on one occasion; fortunately their home is not mine. The next day they were abnormally interested, but no longer sceptical, unless they were just too tired to argue.

> *'My wife has had a remarkable recovery from long standing arthritis of the hip, and an index finger which has been affected for years is now quite flexible (this in 10 days).' Testimonial 124.*

> *'. . . . but it was when I saw a letter my relative sent me, telling of a man who had waited for a hip operation for 2½ years, after taking Feverfew (I don't know for how long) his orthopaedic surgeon said 'no need for the operation.' Testimonial 249.*

> *'. . . . one hand 17 stitches because it almost closed up now I was going to have one on my left one, but since taking one month supply of Feverfew my hand is straightened so I cancelled my op.'*
> *Testimonial 164.*

Regression

Regression can happen, but it is normally due to alcohol, so if you like a drink do make sure that you read the section that deals with alcohol *before* writing to me. Ingestion of drugs for another perhaps temporary malady can also cause temporary loss of benefit.

Average times to benefit; what can I expect to happen, and how long does it take? These are some of the most popular questions, but it simply is not possible to give an accurate assessment for any individual, because of the immense number of combinations available by virtue of differences in physiology. However, if you are not going to be too pernickety I can quote averages, but *please* do remember that they are averages within a timescale that has wandered between immediately and 3 months on occasion in cases of arthritis.

1. To relief from the majority of pain .... 7 days
2. To relief from soreness, swelling and inflammation .... 14 days
3. To remarked improvement (mobility) .... 14–28 days

I am normally unwilling to quote averages, because, despite what I say, people will always take them as personal targets and be upset if they don't apply. Pointers 1–3 are simply an indication of what the average person may expect if the system is clear of drugs, and if good quality *herbal* tablets of the optimum dosage, of fresh leaf from the correct variety of Feverfew, are used—all other things being equal, which in accordance with Sod's Law (what can go wrong will do so, usually at the worst moment) they rarely are.

> *'To my amazement within an hour or so my elbows were free from pain. I couldn't believe. I was squeezing my elbows and had to tell someone so I told 2 complete strangers next to me . . . unbelievable.'*
> *Testimonial 184.*

Tut, Tut. Such unseemly behaviour, but you can't really blame her, for pre-Feverfew she had been unable to carry home the shopping without a great deal of pain.

> *'You will be pleased to know that my sister is delighted with the relief from pain in her hands. She looks at her hands and says that it is a miracle that so much of the swelling has*

gone down. The times you gave for relief from pain, and reduction in swelling were very near.'
Testimonial 209.

Now that trials have been carried out on humans for a change, what may we expect Feverfew to do for animal-kind? Just the same as it happens, but do refer to the dosage section. There is nothing funny about watching a dog chasing your precious cat up the garden path, especially when the dog could hardly walk a few weeks earlier.

'At that time my West Highland Terrier had developed arthritis in one back leg and she was pretty miserable . . . inevitable injections and pills with no good result. So I wrote away for Feverfew tablets and within a week or so there was a decided "lightening of the spirit" as you say, and within a few weeks she was chasing squirrels, and was able to jump onto my bed again (worse luck).'
Testimonial 42.

There are many testimonials concerning animals in my collection. I do urge you to read numbers 283 and 284 where our equine friends are included.

Migraine

I don't know much about migraine except that it is very painful. We talk about the crippling effects of arthritis, but migraine is also crippling. My dictionary says that cripple means disable or impair, and who would be prepared to argue that migraine does not disable or impair? How else can we define an ailment that causes people to shut themselves away in darkened rooms, sometimes for days at a stretch, the mere possibility of light or noise being a a terrifying prospect?

What causes migraine? Apart from the sinus congestion aspect of migraine I think that nobody really knows, because if the cause were known I am sure that a synthetic cure would have been made available long since. It is not only an illness of modern times; some would have us believe that the speed of modern living is the cause. The speed of modern living would not have been the cause in the Middle Ages, but they knew migraine, and they knew trauma.

I am not sufficiently conversant with the different types of migraine to attempt a technical breakdown, but in truth I feel that such a breakdown would be out of place in this book, for it might indicate that different treatments would be necessary. This is not the case, for all migraine responds favourably to Feverfew in some degree, whether it be partial or total, temporary or permanent. Those cases that show permanent relief are caused by trauma, and those that appear to have temporary relief are the result of continuing stress. At this stage, I have not broken down which type of migraine is the result of which cause, but any migraine will respond to the herb given the opportunity.

As with arthritis, any resumption of pain will not be the return of the old pain, but a new trauma of stress-induced condition. Some people appear to live in a state of permanent trauma, due entirely to their lifestyles. They wander from crisis to crisis, rarely settling too long in one place, using Feverfew simply as a painkiller. The herb will only kill pain under such conditions; it will not give permanent relief as it will in single trauma-induced migraine.

A letter that arrived recently shows how complicated treatment can be in the case of migraine. On the surface it would appear to be a matter of allergic reaction, but as soon as I read that it had lasted for 18 months I knew that it could not be. The worst case of allergic reaction on record only lasted 1 month, and mildly at that. For this reason I believe that it is better discussed in the migraine section of the book rather than the allergy section.

The lady in question informed me that she had experienced allergic reaction after taking raw leaf without food, although she had taken it with food but without allergy prior to this. This in itself is not unusual because raw leaf coming into direct contact with the mouth quite often leads to allergic reaction. During the 18 months of what the lady thought was allergic reaction, she had received relief from migraine, but she had a permanent bad taste in the mouth, a ridged tongue, and liquid mucous running down the back of her throat. The type of migraine was not stipulated, but the mucous gives a very good indication. Visits to the doctor, a dermatologist, and a dental hospital revealed nothing amiss, except "it sometimes happens to ladies of my age, 60." Another quote from the manual? Even blood tests revealed nothing untoward. So what was really happening?

> *'You probably know, but it is useful for sinus sufferers also.'*
> *Testimonial 108.*

Yes, I do know because a number of people have told me, but as with other ailments in Group 2, people seem to take relief for granted whilst shouting to the Heavens about the relief from the pain of arthritis. Well, sinus relief is just as important to a lot of people, so do write and tell me about it, and that way it should soon graduate to Group 1. Membership in either group depends on the number of votes cast, so don't think because you have cast a vote for arthritis that you may not vote for something else.

Back to my lady; I am surprised that the implications of the mucous escaped her, but she goes on to say.

> *'1. I definitely had fewer migraines, and those I had were milder..*
> *2. I feel tempted should they increase again to take the tablets that are now available.' Testimonial 159.*

It is unlikely that this lady will have to take Feverfew again because in my opinion she falls into the same category as those people who derive permanent relief from migraine from Day 1. The herb is working superefficiently for her, but I wish that her introduction had been through tablet form; the fresh leaf appears to have overstimulated her sinus relief, and I am more interested at present in slowing down the reaction, which I believe will be possible with the use of fresh orange juice.

It might be thought that I have done the cause of Feverfew a disservice by quoting this letter, but this book has not been written in order to persuade you to run to the nearest shop to buy a preparation of Feverfew. What I am attempting to do is to give you the whole picture, not only as I see it, but as it is seen through the eyes of so many people qualified by experience, not only of Feverfew, but of synthetic drugs as well.

It may be seen from the testimonials that many people claim to have tried just about every drug on the market over a period of years, and admit that one or two have given a degree of relief before being withdrawn, but none has given relief without noticeable side-effects. Certainly, no synthetic drug is recorded as having given the relief that Feverfew has given, without adverse side-effects. What period of relief from migraine would you as an individual require to convince you that the relief might be permanent? Would it be a month, six months, a year perhaps? It is all relative, isn't it? If you have had thrice weekly migraine, relief for one month might appear miraculous; if only one migraine per month, you would require proof over at least six months, maybe even more, if you are difficult to convince.

You may be inclined to believe that by talking about permanent relief I am trying to convince you that you will not have a migraine again. But I repeat what I said earlier; the next migraine would have to come from a different cause if you are trauma induced; it would not come as a result of a previous trauma, and you would, therefore, need to repeat a course of Feverfew treatment.

My definition of permanent is that given by testimonials. The following will give you a reasonable idea of what you may expect in this respect.

> *'It is 7 months since I started taking Feverfew, and as well as relief from arthritis my migraine is almost a thing of the past.'*
> *Testimonial 7.*

> *'. . . . after suffering for many years from severe attacks of migraine. The relief was indescribable when my attacks became less frequent, and it is now more than 2 years since I had an attack.'*
> *Testimonial 8.*

> *'A cousin of mine who suffered from migraine for years finds complete relief by taking leaves each morning, and it has cured her for car sickness; she has been a chronic sufferer from childhood.'*
> *Testimonial 20.*

> *'I have found it most beneficial in the relief of migraine from which I have suffered all my life.'*
> *Testimonial 37.*

> *'I already take it when in need for migraine, which I have found very good results.'*
> *Testimonial 65.*

There is much to be learned from these 5 testimonials. In 7 and 20 we can see that the treatment is continuous, in one case for at least 7 months, in the other for a period of years. This is not the correct way to take Feverfew, for once the herb has done its work there is no necessity to continue treatment. These two cases appear to be trauma-induced, so relief following a proper course should be permanent requiring minimum top-up—if any. Number 8 is very typical in the progressive relief gained, and claims permanent final relief. Unfortunately, it does not specify if treatment is continuing or at what stage it ceased, or the frequency of attacks. Be that as it may the lady is obviously delighted, and 2 years should be sufficient to convince any sceptic, although longer periods have been claimed.

In common with many, testimonial 7 claims relief from two Group 1 ailments, but I get the impression that the arthritis was the primary concern, with migraine being accepted as a beneficial side-effect.

Number 20 details one Group 1 ailment and one Group 2. Number 37 is rather vague because it tells us only that relief has been obtained. It does not tell us the degree of severity or frequency, or the duration of treatment.

Testimonial 65 is a prime example of how not to use Feverfew as a simple painkiller. I know that it may be used in this way, but this is not its primary function. Although the Feverfew is efficient, and only a small amount is required to give benefit, it is imperative that the body should be given sufficient amounts during an intensive course for it to be able to get to the root of the trouble. We know that individual requirements vary, so the only way to ensure that a reservoir is available is to take the herb until benefit is received, then either reduce the intake progressively, or cease treatment; I prefer reducing the intake.

Number 65 also misses the point relative to the full benefit that Feverfew bestows; by using the herb as a painkiller this lady still has to brace herself for each successive attack. By the correct use of Feverfew she can remove this potentially harmful period of anticipatory stress, which in each attack of migraine is an aggravatory problem.

I said earlier that Feverfew is intended basically to give long-term relief, and that remains my personal view, but I cannot dictate how you should use the herb. The following example is typical, but the herb is being used simply to support a lifestyle that does not suit the individual concerned.

> *'A friend of mine sent me a copy of your broadsheet, and after reading it I decided to give Feverfew a try. . . . The change in my life is remarkable, no longer dominated by stress-caused headaches. . . . I would recommend Feverfew to all migraine sufferers without a doubt. . . . I lead a very hectic life which probably caused my migraine. It is lovely to be able to dash around without the fear of one coming on. Your broadsheet saved me. Thank you.'*
> *Testimonial 279.*

I don't think I have done this lady a favour by helping to perpetuate a life of stressful activity, I would rather help her realize that she is being given a warning by the stress-induced migraine. I had not intended to introduce stress-induced migraine at this point because it is more relevant to other ailments and complementary to them, but this last testimonial does serve as an object lesson. If migraines continue after a course of Feverfew, don't blame the herb before you have taken a long hard look at your way of life. Don't kid yourself, be honest and if you can see that your life consists of a daily series of trauma, the remedy for the most part lies in your own hands. The herb will help you to overcome the stress, but you will be very lucky if even Feverfew will help to the degree that it has helped the lady of testimonial 279.

In this section, I have dealt with trauma-induced migraine, and as you have seen it is very possible that you will gain permanent relief if your problem is of this nature. If having gained relief for a period of years you are again subjected to attacks, please regard two things—either you have undergone a recent traumatic experience, or you have changed your lifestyle and introduced stress-induced migraine.

Psoriasis

There has been more scepticism in respect to psoriasis than any of the Group 1 ailments, and I believe that the reason is that there is no oral medication given in orthodox medicine. I am aware of the oral supplement to ultra-violet treatment, but this is a totally different matter. This supplementary treatment is given in order to ensure thorough saturation of the skin, and has no other value. Doctors are reluctant to use this oral factor because of known side-effects.

Precisely what is psoriasis? The *Encyclopedia Brittanica* defines it as a chronic, recurrent skin disorder, characterised by reddish, slightly raised placques or papules (solid elevations) covered with silvery-white scales. In most cases, says *Brittanica,* the lesions tend to be symmetrically distributed on the elbows and knees, scalp, chest and buttocks.

I am most surprised that feet, legs and hands are not mentioned, and if we include these why not simply say that it may affect the entire body? Further information from this same source tells us that the nails are frequently involved, becoming thickened, irregularly laminated and brittle.

We are also told that the cause of psoriasis is not known, but that the lesions are believed to result from abnormalities in both the novascular horny layers of the outer skin and its deeper vascular layer. It is reported to affect between 1 and 2% of the white population of northern climates, and it is believed that rheumatoid arthritis is a direct consequence of psoriasis.

What can we say about that? The cause is unknown, but we are expected to believe that another major ailment is a direct consequence of the ailment. I realize, of course, that my case is hypothetical, but having seen not only one ailment derive benefit from Feverfew, but 2, 3 and even 4 at the same time, I am inclined to believe that the hypothesis is nearer the truth than even I am prepared to admit at present. If we can accept that testimonials are true and given in good faith, we have an anomaly; hypothesis supported by fact. You may argue of course that my case is only hypothetical in respect of the primary function of the herb, and not in respect of the cures which are self-evident. I accept that, and admit that my primary consideration is to set people talking, discussing and evaluating. While this is being done there is always the chance that combined research may be stated, in an attempt to discover the common factor that links together my Group 1 ailments.

In the 1970s, reports on novel methods and medications in the treatment of psoriasis were numerous, but there was no generally effective cure. At this point I willingly acknowledge my debt to *Brittanica,* for it has been a very useful tool, not only for my work, but for the rest of the family in various projects over the past few years. This does not necessarily mean that I have to consider myself bound by the opinion contained therein, and in this respect I did not consult this mini-library until my personal opinions were well and truly formulated. It would have been only too easy to get off on the wrong foot if I had read the opinions of other people earlier. As a result I was most surprised when I finally opened the books and discovered precisely how little is known about the Group 1 ailments.

The Birmingham Trials mentioned earlier would appear to support the view expressed in *Brittanica* that rheumatoid arthritis is a consequence of psoriasis, but I contend that the arthritis was already present, latent perhaps and virtually unnoticed, but still present. Creaky knees are a sign of age to many people and would not necessarily be regarded as symptomatic of the presence of arthritis. My theories are entirely based on a common imbalance, which has as its symptoms any combination of Group 1 ailments. The excess of substances in the blood that are responsible for these symptoms may reveal themselves in severe arthritis plus mild psoriasis, mild arthritis with total heavy coverage of psoriasis, or many points in between, and there is also the coincidence of migraine to take into account.

As I see it then, once the imbalance has begun it is the individual metabolic reaction that dictates the course of events, resulting in perhaps a single but very noticeable manifestation of one ailment, with accompanying slight effects of the remainder of Group 1 ailments, excluding migraine, or it may encourage an even distribution of effect involving a combination of imbalance. I fully accept the coincidence of effect in one person of single and multiple symptoms, and I believe that after reading the following testimonials, you will agree that there is substance in this belief. At the very least they should encourage support of my theory that psoriasis may not be considered in isolation any more, but that it should be taken in context with arthritis and migraine.

> *'I should like to mention that as seems normal, I too suffer not only with migraine but also have a touch of arthritis (in a not too severe form as yet), and have an allergy to heat such that I get a touch of psoriasis on the elbows, also small itchy blisters on the hands in hot weather or when I have been unfortunate enough to have a temperature.'*
> *Testimonial 71.*

> *'I suffer from arthritis and psoriasis, and it is the latter that I am most concerned about. I eat a couple of leaves twice a day (plant permitting) and find it is helping to clear it.'*
> *Testimonial 152.*

> *'I have been for 20 years a psoriasis sufferer. Doctors, Specialists, Faith Healers, Hypnosis, all have failed, but after one week of Feverfew the irritation has gone and now the patches have diminished, the soreness gone and the discoloration fading.'*
> *Testimonial 168.*

> *'For your information the Feverfew is helping a great deal with the perpetual headaches I used to suffer from. . . . far less frequent. With regard to the (sorry I cannot spell it) skin rash, this was never very bad, and was brought on by heat, and this summer was very hot but I had no sign of it. P.S. I started noticing a beneficial effect within 2 or 3 days.'*
> *Testimonial 227.*

'I have been taking Feverfew for over a year now, and find that I seldom get a migraine, and if I do it is much milder than before, and I do not get the sickness with the migraine like I used to. Also I used to get psoriasis very badly on my knees and elbows, also odd places on my body but since taking Feverfew, this has all cleared up.'
Testimonial 277.

'I suffered with rheumatism in my toes, and could only walk short distances, without resting. I also had psoriasis on my head. After three days I noticed a distinct improvement with the rheumatism. I can now walk in complete comfort and the patches on my head are much improved.'
Testimonial 265.

If I could only offer the last six testimonials in support of my theory regarding the link that has been established between arthritis, migraine and psoriasis, I should be able to excuse the cynics who even now will be girding up their loins ready to have me for breakfast. This is not the case, I am delighted to say, for you have only to study the testimonials at the back of the book to find many more. Quite sufficient for many people to agree that while I may not be 100 % right, I am getting somewhere near, and that is the object of the exercise.

Do these last six testimonials have special points of interest for us? Well, 71 is an example of the tripartite agreement between Group 1 ailments. The psoriasis is of the heat-aggravated stress-induced variety for the most part, but it is of the long standing trauma-induced variety in the case of the elbows. Both types respond well to Feverfew. 265 tells of an improvement in scalp psoriasis, and in my experience this is the most difficult to deal with as well as the most potentially embarrassing. 277 highlights the point I made earlier regarding the omission from *Brittanica* regarding feet and legs, for while feet in particular have not played a major part in my research concerning psoriasis, they have appeared in cases of total coverage. I feel that it would be true to say that feet are related to dense total coverage, to be specific.

Between 1 and 2 % of the white population of northern latitudes represents a considerable number of people, and it naturally only includes those people who have consulted a doctor. Many have not, considering it to be merely a heat rash. I would not like to hazard a guess at the true number, but I have come across many who had no idea what the condition was. It was simply a seasonal problem, a minor upset that wasn't worth getting steamed up about, but all the same they have been pleased when it disappeared along with migraine or arthritis.

I mentioned briefly the effect of psoriasis on daily life, and it is perfectly obvious that it does have a stressful effect on those afflicted, both men and women. On one occasion, I came across a man who would not even leave another room to speak to me, so embarrassed was he, and it must be more embarrassing for women. Men can get away with a lot in this respect, but not so women. I believe that the medical profession recognizes the stress associated with this complaint, but there is little they can do except to issue tranquilizers, and we all know what that leads to.

To date no failures have been reported concerning the effect of Feverfew on psoriasis; this does not mean that there have been none. So if you have a case of failure to report, don't worry about hurting my feelings. I am not in the game of white-washing Feverfew; I want to know it all, but I do ask you to recall what I said at the beginning of this section: it has been stubborn and you must be patient. Sometimes relief begins within days, but one case of total coverage took 6 months. Remember when you write that I need facts not fantasies. I don't want to hear that you think there has been an improvement. I want only facts, and by writing to me you may be able to help millions of other people. This is not an exaggeration; the most surprising tests have set off new lines of research.

One of the cases involved in the research of psoriasis was an elderly gentleman, and I asked him why he was trying Feverfew. He said that there was nowhere else to go, he had tried everything else. I looked at him and couldn't fail to notice the twinkle in his eye. I told him to have patience—just as well that he holds the record for the longest time spent in total clearance, 6 months. I do not want a new record holder. Six months is long enough even if you have had the problem for 100 years.

Stress

Such a little word for so great a problem; you could be forgiven for thinking that it should stretch across a page, but stress is in at the beginning, the middle and the end of so many illnesses. If it is not responsible for starting them, it is most certainly responsible for the aggravation of many. Asthma springs readily to mind in this respect.

While I am quietly confident that trauma will eventually be recognized as the villain of the piece as far as Group 1 at least is concerned, I must make it perfectly clear that I do differentiate between trauma and stress.

Since I have used these terms extensively throughout the book, it might be as well if I explained my interpretation of them.

I define trauma as sudden, short, sharp shock, a once only effect in connection with a specific incident. Amazingly enough as I took a break from working on this book, precisely at this point in the manuscript, I read in the Letters column of a daily newspaper about a lady who claimed that she had developed agoraphobia after receiving a shock whilst dismounting from a bus 30 years before. This really was amazing because the ailment has very recently come into the sphere of Feverfew, but I have a long way to go with it yet.

Stress I define as continuing trauma of a lesser degree. It is possible for many events in daily life to be traumatic to a person who is tired or run down. Even minor events that would not merit notice in most people's eyes assume monumental proportions to such people, and the usual response given to a request for medication is, of course, yes you've guessed it, tranquilizers. Strangely enough, the body might cope perfectly well with initial trauma, but if stress becomes more than the body can stand; the army of self-repair technicians is overwhelmed, and the problem becomes long term due to the resulting breakdown in communication.

Authors and playwrights mention heart-stopping experiences, and there can be little doubt that severe trauma has been the cause of many sudden deaths. This is the supreme effect of trauma, and while it may be true in the relatively small number of cases, the example shows the extreme effect that trauma can wreak on the human body. If we can accept that the trauma can kill, should we not be equally ready to accept that it can have other effects not quite as dramatic as death, even on a healthy person?

If you do not accept this theory, perhaps you would care to advance another, explaining why a person in seemingly good health should suddenly become affected by arthritis, migraine and psoriasis. I have seen it happen amongst my colleagues. I have a clinical detachment in such situations, but I have often wondered why people do not tell me to mind my own business when I ask if they know the cause. I never have been told to mind my own business, but this may be due to the surprise question, it never having entered the mind of the person concerned that anything caused it, it just happened. I have received many testimonials that confirm the coincidence of trauma with the onset of one or more of the Group 1 ailments.

If somebody has already strung together by common factors those ailments that form the current sphere of involvement of Feverfew, they have kept very quiet about it. There may be good and sufficient reason for this silence, but if it is other than commercial I most certainly have never heard of it, and there are plenty of clinical trials underway for adverse reactions to have been noted. As far as I am concerned information is like dung: to do any good it must be spread around.

You may have wondered why, if I feel that stress is an integral part of other ailments, I have devoted a separate section to it. The reason is that the masses have now accepted that stress is a separate entity, and for this reason I am obliged to put cart before horse again. Why does it exist at all, and how can it maintain a separate identity? It exists simply because the affected mind is not in receipt of the data necessary for corrective influence to be exerted, or because if the information is available it is not getting through. I know that I have mentioned this before in other contexts, but it is here that the problem is at its most formidable. It is entirely possible for the mind to reach such a state prior to correction that a normal state is virtually impossible to achieve, and we are then right over the top.

Talk is cheap, and I would not blame you for thinking that a bus inspector can have but little knowledge of the real meaning of deep stress. For this reason I am going to quote an example in which I have been personally involved, in the hope that you will then understand that I am in fact no stranger to this factor.

My experience of stress involved a young man. At university he succumbed to pre-examination nerves and was intent on committing suicide. He was prevented by classmates from so doing, and he was returned to his family for out-patient treatment.

His case was desperate, and it was most distressing to watch such a fine young man deteriorate into a vegetable. His life was regulated by his drug calendar, and this was his only response throughout long lonely days, except for an occasional meal. It was exceptional to receive a response to a greeting when I visited him with my wife. Suppressant drugs, given to prevent further attempts at suicide, had reduced him to this state, but there was certainly no progress towards normality.

All else having failed, he was scheduled to enter a local hospital which specialized in such problems, but within two weeks prior to admission it was made possible for him to be placed in the care of my wife and myself. His parents were worn out, and we cudgelled them into taking a holiday that had been booked long before. They didn't want to go, and even at the airport they contemplated a return.

The following week was the nearest thing to Hell on earth that my wife and I are likely to experience. We were determined to win him back. When I say that plans had been made I do not mean detailed plans, for I am ever conscious of Sod's Law, and the best plans are always basically simple. I have seen too many chains break because of a weak link, and what you can drop into on such occasions can be far from pleasant.

My contribution to the effort was to surprise but interest him. So I stripped down his car engine and set him to polishing bits and pieces. That surprised him, I can tell you, and he developed a sudden interest in getting it back together again; we did 3 engines in 9 days; the only casualty was the bottom end of his own engine when we increased the power at the top, but the cost was worth his deep belly laugh. Meanwhile my wife got him back to former interests—jigsaw puzzles, crosswords, etc.—and kept him constructively busy in her allotted time while I was at work.

It was the end of the first week before he realized that he had not taken any sedatives or sleeping tablets. We had not deliberately withheld them; we simply forgot to remind him, and he was sleeping so deeply because of his labours that it seemed such a pity to awaken him. At the end of that fortnight he was pronounced fit, subject only to a week's holiday to return to college. His parents telephoned from the airport on their return to ask how he was, so off he went in his car to pick them up.

End of story? Not quite; two years later he asked to see the witch doctors again, but it took only a few hours. This man is now a highly trained engineer; he has a lovely wife and family, and he commutes internationally on a regular basis. He lives a lifestyle that would kill me, but his confidence is such that he lives life to the full. Only my wife and I know what the fortnight cost us, but it was worth every moment and we thank God that we had the strength. He did it and so can you.

We had looked closely at the so-called borders of insanity—the thin line that divides the world most of us know from a darker, unplumbed world, only an incident or set of circumstances away. Can it really be so? The journey into such a state may be only a moment away, of terribly short duration. In certain circumstances the mind plays weird tricks, and a state of fantasy may become infinitely preferable to reality. Is insanity a response to trauma? Most certainly, but the effect does not have to appear so obvious. Take agoraphobia, for instance. It is a response to a traumatic situation, but it could so easily have been channelled into a Group 1 ailment or combination of ailments; the body has simply worked through a different channel. The answer is still the same: find the point of selective affinity.

As my mail bag grows larger I wonder at the depth of Feverfew involvement. I can tell you only a little of what I know because there are too many people ready to scoff that I am offering a panacea for all ills. They will learn the hard way, possibly, because one or two have already succumbed to some of the ailments mentioned, and it has been a case of swallowing pride and the bitter Feverfew pill, all else having failed. I have been fortunate in coming into contact with some individuals who appear to be quite enlightened. I don't mean that they accept everything I say, but they are prepared to look into it and they do have the facilities and influence to make their presence felt.

How do we know that Feverfew is effective in dissimilar areas of stress?

> *'In 1969 I began taking the contraceptive pill, and within 6 months I had my first migraine attack.'*
> *Testimonial 31.*

> *'1. My aches and pains for the arthritis have improved.*
> *2. Trouble with migraine has vanished.*
> *3. Menopausal problems have improved.'*
> *Testimonial 137.*

> *'I have had arthritis since I was 16, I am now 35 . . . I had also suffered migraine since my second child was born, I had weekly attacks. After three days of taking the tablets the arthritic pain has gone and I have not had a migraine since. I have not been so free of pain for years.'*
> *Testimonial 192.*

An interesting combination, don't you think, but consider them and form your own conclusions as to which problem is the result of stress, or trauma, or both.

Premenstrual tension

Without a doubt, premenstrual tension is one of the major problems encountered in some degree by the majority of fertile women. Unfortunately, it is treated lightly by some G.P.'s because it appears to involve only a few days each month, but this is a fallacy. I do not consider it lightly, nor do I say "you will have to put up with it" because it is a serious problem, involving quite a slice of each woman's month. First is the anticipation, then the period itself, followed by a state of mental unrest until the effect wears off. How much of the month does that leave? Not a great deal by my reckoning. Even if I have quoted the worst case it is not an impossible case, and a lot of women will agree with me. But I do not expect them to believe the next part of the text any more than I expect the majority of people to believe it.

The monthly period is a regular provocation for the fertile woman whether she realizes it or not; career women or those who have deliberately chosen to put off starting a family are prone to sense it, like it or not. A chemical imbalance occurs and no automatic remedial action is taken because the brain does not have the data to base reaction.

Can you now accept this precept? If you can, I suggest that as your next period approaches you should consider what I have said in this context, and I feel sure that the problem will be lessened. Only you can put the data into the old brain box. If you need a little help for a couple of months until you get used to it, Feverfew will help. Culpeper and Gerard used it a lot in similar cases, and they always regarded it as *the herb for women*.

Menopause

Many women in menopause are still concerned with reproduction, and they fear that the future no longer holds the promise of fulfillment. You would be surprised at the number of women who have told me that they feel less womanly for this lack, that they are letting their partner down because they can no longer bear children. I have spoken to too many women at this stage of life not to be able to discern the cause of a fear that appears not to have a foundation; they feel terrible but can't tell you why.

Once again we have a chemical imbalance that should be corrected automatically if the brain knew its job or could get the message through. It is necessary to acknowledge the cause of this mental upset before the brain can get to work. Feverfew helps in these circumstances by relieving the stress caused by the anxiety, leaving you to cope with the basic problem. It will lighten your spirit and give you a bit of get-up-and-go, so get on with it. No more moping.

Supplementary treatments can be given at this time, but the majority of doctors are unwilling to use them—wisely I believe—not only because of known side-effects, but also because if the body suddenly starts to do its own correction, nasty things could happen. As a problem it has been with us for some time, but it is well within the powers of human physiology to correct this imbalance naturally. It is sometimes a problem deciding whether trauma is wholly to blame, or whether stress is partially to blame.

Look again at testimonial 137 and you will see what I mean, because it is a very interesting combination of cause, effect and treatment. You may have already decided where the blame should lie as regards cause, but one fact is clear: treatment is standard. Feverfew has given benefit in all three cases, and the cause is of academic interest only.

Now we come to a point in the story that fascinates me and is the point at which light begins to appear at the end of the tunnel. I am satisfied that the link between arthritis, migraine and psoriasis is sufficiently proven as regards effect and possibly even cause, i.e., trauma or stress, but between the two lies a grey area. What is the actual effect of the cause in terms of chemical imbalance?

In the cases of arthritis, migraine and stress we have been considering over-production of inflammatory substances, and we have observed the regulatory effect of Feverfew, but in menopause, whilst still observing the regulatory effect, we are seeing the other side of the coin. The tap is opening to permit greater flow of the necessary corrective chemicals, chiefly estrogen. In fertile women, i.e., before the onset of menopause, this hormone is produced in two areas of the body; the reproductive function is supplied in the main by the ovaries, while the balance of estrogen required for the remainder of bodily functions is supplied by the adrenal gland.

There it is again, the adrenal gland. In scrutinizing the effects of research in connection with arthritis, we have seen that Paul Hench obtained his compound E from the cortex of the adrenal gland, and this has been sufficient for me to take a closer look at this particular area. This is not because I really want to know the effect of compound E or estrogen alone (they have already been catalogued sufficiently); but because we now have two significant substances emerging from the same area, involving two apparently unrelated ailments, both yielding to Feverfew.

Have we reached a point of selective affinity? Maybe, but more proof is needed before I could accept that this is the case. I would need to be able to indicate other substances derived from the same area, having been proven to be a shortfall in other ailments that I accept as being within the sphere of activity of the herb. I have not read anywhere that we can attribute arthritis to estrogen excess or deficiency, or hot flashes to incorrect levels of compound E.

I assume that estrogen levels are measurable in the same way that it is possible to measure the excess of prostaglandins in the case of arthritis. If I am right, then it should be a relatively simple matter to compare the estrogen levels pre- and post-Feverfew in a woman experiencing menopausal problems. A relationship would be possible then between levels established post-Feverfew and what would be considered the norm for a woman in what could be considered desirable menopause, i.e., without the problems experienced by 50% of women at this period of life.

H.R.T. is a treatment for menopausal problems, but instead of being simply an estrogen-only supplement, it is now a combination of two substances, estrogen and progesterone (or its synthetic equivalent, Progestogen). This combination was made necessary by the unfortunate side-effects of the estrogen-only supplement and many explain why even today doctors are loath to prescribe H.R.T.

I believe that Feverfew can boost the production of an estrogen-based combination that brings the supply necessary for normal bodily functions during the period of stress up to a required level. At the same time the female body is adjusting to the loss of the reproductive function and the loss of supplies from the ovaries, which may or may not have been taken up solely by this function.

One postmenopausal effect is osteoporosis, although this problem is not confined to women or to the postmenopausal period. Why should I believe that Feverfew could apply to this ailment? I have no proof; therefore what I can say on the subject is mere supposition. I have faith in Feverfew, and in taking a closer look at osteoporosis I have noted that it appears to be directly or indirectly related to estrogen deficiency. Osteoporosis is a softening or weakening of bone tissue and often the cause of an apparent reduction in height, or excessive stooping in older people. So I offer a further test. Is it possible to evaluate relative calcium acceptance or levels between a victim of osteoporosis, and someone accepting calcium normally and making normal use of it? Tests showing relative levels in the afflicted person pre- and post-Feverfew could be revealing; in fact I am prepared to say they *would* be revealing.

I'm sure that you will now appreciate my excitement at the relationship of arthritis and menopause both through effect in reaction to Feverfew, and by the coincidence of the area from which the problem associated with both appear to have their origin. I do not pretend that the adrenal glands, estrogen and compound E hold the final answer, just as I do not accept that the effect of Feverfew on the control of prostaglandins is a final answer, they are but steps on the way. Feverfew knows the answer and is proving extraordinarily loath to give up the secret, but what a fascinating quest. I can easily understand now how people can immerse themselves in research to the exclusion of all else.

GROUP 2

Fringe benefits

The effects of Feverfew on the ailments mentioned thus far, with one or two exceptions that have been used as examples only, have all been adequately proven by testimonial. The testimonials at the back of the book have been selected because they have a little bit extra to say, but they are only a portion of those that arrived during the six months prior to the writing of this book. I have not bothered to count the total, but they are many. Those undergoing both long- and short-term treatment to assess the effects of Feverfew should be aware that the herb continues to give benefit long after ingestion has ceased.

In Group 2 ailments without exception the testimonials have mentioned improvement as a beneficial side-effect gained whilst treatment has been undertaken for another ailment. As I said earlier they have not graduated to Group 1 as yet because so far I consider them to be not proven. However, testimonials arrive daily, and there is no reason to suppose that they will not be up there. This is the fascination of Feverfew: just when I think that I have arrived at the end of the road, something new pops up and sets me off again.

At present the medical establishment is becoming more and more prepared to accept Feverfew for relief of migraine, but there is a long way to go before they will accept it for arthritis, and even further for psoriasis, so what chance do Group 2 ailments stand at present?

This book, as it stands at present, owes two things only to medical research: the effect on the white cells and the fact that to date nothing adverse has been discovered. No part of it has yet received medical agreement apart from these two points.

Incontinence

Would you disagree that apart from certain external influences incontinence is the result of stress? It is certainly my contention that it is, especially in the long term, in which case trauma is not responsible.

Shock will cause this effect in the shorter term, mainly as a result of continuing stress. As the problem gets to a certain stage, embarrassment steps in to ensure that the problem becomes even more stressful and therefore more embarrassing, and so a vicious circle is brought into being.

> *'. . . . but to me the great benefit of Feverfew is that I don't get waterworks trouble. I was taking xxxxxx tablets and after a year I was getting pain when I passed water, was going to the toilet approximately every 30 minutes or less . . . I got to the stage where I could not get home from work without leaving a train, going to the toilet, and catching the next one; was up 12-14 times each night . . .'*
> *Testimonial 240.*

If you can imagine anything more stressful than this I must hear of it. The embarrassment of pain may be readily understood, because the outward signs are normally visible and even if they are not, nobody minds admitting that a leg or an arm is acting up, but this does not apply to incontinence. Each time a situation arises outside the office or home it is a potential acute embarrassment and a stress inducer. Add to this the problem of having to go to the toilet 12-14 times each night and you have the makings of a fine old mental state. The letter goes on to say:

> *'. . . . within a few short weeks of taking Feverfew my waterworks improved very much, and at the moment although not back as they were, to me excellent.'*

He does not claim a complete cure, but he is satisfied after a few short weeks. I have no doubt that I shall hear more from this gentleman, and I hope that in his next letter he will be all the way back to normal.

Blood pressure

It is a matter of record passed on in testimonials that Feverfew does reduce high blood pressure to a point at or very near normal, but there has been no indication that it reduces the pressure below normal. There have, however, been two reports of palpitations occuring when Feverfew was taken concurrently with high dosage blood pressure tablets. I am pleased to say that no problems have been reported in connection with low dosage blood pressure tablets, and while I am confident that Feverfew will do the job equally well, I have always made a point of advising people with heart problems to have a good chat with the doctor *before* taking Feverfew.

I have only one report that the herb is being taken solely for a blood pressure problem and this from a gentleman who is body and soul against synthetics.

Do please take my advice about seeing your doctor first before taking the herb. I am sure that the majority of doctors will cooperate, but in any event do not simply discard prescribed medicine. If you want your doctor to act responsibly towards you, you must reciprocate.

> *'My head feels a lot clearer now (I have high blood pressure) and I am beginning to take an interest in life again, before this I felt like a zombie.'*
> *Testimonial 343.*

> *'May I say how much Feverfew has helped me in one month; my arthritis has ceased and my blood pressure is down.'*
> *Testimonial 329.*

Fingernails

This effect really was interesting, especially since before opening *Brittanica* I had tended to regard it as a lonely soldier. Now of course, having gathered my scattered wits and looked again at the testimonials that mention the problem, it becomes quite clear. Like mud, you say. I cannot say that fingernails are a problem only when there are other signs of the presence of psoriasis. It would not be true. But since it is purported to be a manifestation of psoriasis in its own right, I am not surprised to discover it to be in concert with other Group 1 ailments.

> *'A further benefit is that my fingernails which were extremely brittle are now stronger, and do not grow at such a rapid rate as before.' Testimonial 292.*

> *'I feel much brighter and not so dopey. I have also noticed an improvement in my fingernails which do not flake as they did.' Testimonial 300.*

> *'For many years since the birth of our son over 30 years ago she has suffered from continual splitting of the finger-*

nail. On all her fingers the nail split almost down to the quick, which has been rather painful as well as inconvenient. However, since she started taking Feverfew tablets most of the splitting has stopped.' Testimonial 237.

Hayfever, asthma, cat and dog allergy, general irritants

All in one? Yes, there is one testimonial at the back that deals with the whole bundle except asthma. Testimonial 239. It is in detail at the back, so just turn to it when you feel like it. I don't mind.

Once again I admit to surprise when this grouping came up, but with the benefit of hindsight and brain in gear it has to be logical. The major problem with many such ailments is soreness and inflammation. If the herb relieves sinus congestion, there is no reason why it should not relieve soreness and inflammation in the same area. In fact for all I know that is how it relieves sinus problems.

Hayfever is definitely related because of the effect of the herb on sore and inflamed areas, either membrane in the nose or passages in the throat. I don't know if controlled release of compound E is involved, but it it isn't I shall be surprised.

Cat, dog and general allergy appear to be unlikely bedfellows, but the effect on the person is similar to the effect of hayfever, and as seems to be the case. Feverfew will help in these ailments too. This does not in any way invalidate my basic theory. It merely indicates that the Work Centre in which Feverfew does its work is more widely responsible than I had previously thought. It is possible that the sphere of involvement will continue to grow, but the ailments will share the common factors of stress or trauma as a cause, soreness, swelling and inflammation as symptoms.

Hearing

Hearing problems are one of the most unlikely of the ailments that derive benefit from Feverfew. The benefit is given not by direct action of Feverfew on the ear, but by relief of pressure caused by arthritis of the neck. It is a matter of record by testimonial that the herb may help in such cases, but I must stress that there has been no notification of benefit being received if arthritis of the neck is not involved. This is a bit of a tricky situation really, because some people will immediately jump to the conclusion that their hearing problems are due to arthritis and rush out to buy Feverfew.

'Five years ago I also went deaf, and have used a hearing aid for the last few months. This last week, my hearing began to improve, and it had not occurred to me that its cause could be the arthritis in my neck. I am not imagining my improved hearing.'
Testimonial 45.

I am quite prepared to accept that the lady has derived benefit, although she appears to think that I am going to be sceptical. It was certainly a surprise package, but nonetheless welcome for that. I find that I can readily accept it simply because there is a logical explanation. The effects of an arthritic neck are plain to see, and I cannot dream up good and sufficient reason why it should not affect hearing.

Remember, however, that there is no reason to suppose that because Feverfew has helped this lady, it will help you. Your case could be entirely different. If you are completely sure that your hearing has become impaired since you contracted arthritis of the neck, Feverfew may help in this respect.

Eyesight

Now I can hear you say he has really gone over the top this time. Scoff if you like, but nobody was more skeptical than I when the first letter arrived. Not that I didn't believe the lady. She knows better than anyone what has happened to her, but in this case I could not apply logic. Throughout my work I have stuck to this principle; however unlikely, if logic dictates that it is possible, I will spend time on it. Not because I am desperate for something to do, but because it may lead to something else.

So I wrote to thank the lady and then put the letter on one side. No avenue of research is ever entirely closed once opened, but eyesight and hearing are terribly specialized subjects and as such are best left to specialists.

It would have been easy to forget that this side-effect existed, but then along came letter number 2 and the case was brought into the limelight again. Still logic dictated that there was no connection, but the impossible can happen. I stress once again, as with deafness, that I have confined my research in this respect to problems that have begun or worsened *since* the onset of arthritis. My work is not directed at any other area. The point has been made, however, and must be proven or rejected; it cannot be left in thin air. I have accepted it simply because it is a fact in some cases, so I must attempt to prove it, or at the very least offer a reasonable explanation.

Try as might I could not discover a suitable chemical imbalance, and in truth I wasted too much time searching. In other words, I developed tunnel vision. I fell too readily into the trap of making an assumption and then seeking to prove it, wading through reams of paper trying to make something fit. After almost drowning in a sea of information, I pulled myself up by my braces and opened up the vision again to wide angle.

This time I laid out the possible alternatives and went through them one by one. The third alternative was a purely mechanical problem, similar to deafness, but how could the solution be mechanical when there appeared to be no connection? But there is. The six muscles that are responsible for controlling focus in each eye are directed by input from the brain, via semicircular canals in the inner ear, so what effect would arthritis of the neck have upon these channels? Is there a deforming influence exerted by the arthritis that causes improper or inefficient focusing? I put these questions to the experts.

> *'. . . . having bifocals and reading glasses as well, now I can do any close work without the reading glasses and feel so much better generally.'*
> *Testimonial 274.*

> *'I have for some years had my vision marred (not to blindness), but by a kind of black net before my eyes which seemed to dull the vision. . . . I also have arthritis of the neck . . . this was not so bad when taking the leaves, also I woke one morning to find that my sight was much brighter. . . . I can remember my mother going to xxxxx in her later years and they told her it was nothing. . . . she had trouble, her eyes got very sore and she herself maintained it was arthritis. . . .' Testimonial 154.*

Eczema

Is it always called nervous eczema, or are there two types of eczema?

> *'I am an eczema sufferer and as we had a plant in the garden I have been taking the leaves regularly. There has been a marked improvement in my condition.'*
> *Testimonial 188.*

Point taken.

That is quite enough for now about areas of supplementary benefit in connection with the side-effects of treatment by Feverfew. You may well notice other benefits mentioned in the testimonials, and simply because they have not been mentioned in this section of the book this does not mean that I do not accept them. There is a lot of ground between "proven" and "not yet proven" as far as I am concerned, and as I get deeper into my research I find myself trying more and more to comprehend the *modus operandi* of Feverfew. In this respect, more ailments do not make the task more difficult, because eventually I believe that I shall hit on one that has a known point of origin. Once this has been established it should facilitate the task of locating the point of selective affinity.

Allergy

You have been very patient in waiting for me to come to the nitty gritty of allergic reaction, that is, of course, assuming that you have not cheated and taken this section out of turn. You may have had the impression that it is a major problem, but this is not so, except for those unfortunates who cannot use the herb because of allergic reaction, and consequently cannot derive benefit from it.

There is no hard and fast rule by which we can assess potential allergic reaction; it is a fact of life, and at present we must accept it as such. I have tried several methods of combating the effect; so far I have not had success, but I never give up. The incidence of allergy is highest with fresh leaf, at 7%. The effects are mouth ulcers or blisters, a sore throat and itchy skin. This is primary allergy, and it is a comparatively minor effect, as you may have guessed from the fact that my wife voluntarily subjects herself to it if she feels it is justified. It normally lasts between 24 and 72 hours if you cease treatment immediately. There is of course no need for you to have this discomfort if you have had a skin test first, but this test, although it shows that you are allergic to leaf, does not necessarily mean that you are allergic to tablets or capsules.

Skin test

There are two methods to test for allergy to Feverfew, but both naturally involve having a fresh leaf available. The first method is to rub the leaf into the soft skin of the wrist. If you are allergic, an itchy patch will appear within 24 hours and normally disappear as quickly. The second method is to tape a leaf to the wrist with sticking plaster for 24–48 hours, with the same result, but if you choose the second method, do ensure first that you are not allergic to sticking plaster.

So, you have tested and discovered a degree of allergy as far as fresh leaf is concerned, and this means that any contact with the fresh leaf in the mouth would immediately result in the effects mentioned above. The next step is to try the leaf in a small sandwich, and as I have said before, Feverfew should always be taken with food anyway. Never mind that you know somebody who can chew the leaves; they are few and not a good example. If you are one of the few, please don't advise other people to do the same. It could put them off the herb for life if they are squeamish, and many are. They will eat lettuce, but the thought of eating the leaf of a flowering plant—or weed as some prefer to call it—is just too much. Be a good neighbour and tell them the proper way. If you can't think of any, read the testimonials properly; there are plenty of suggestions, or you will find indications from me in the dosage section.

If you find that you are allergic to leaf, don't give up hope. The commercial products available greatly reduce the incidence of allergy, and you may yet be lucky. The best products give the highest incidence of allergy simply because they are closer to the activity levels of fresh leaf, and as these levels of activity decrease so does the incidence of allergy, but it does not disappear altogether. My wife has tried every product we know to be available, and at very low levels of activity the allergic reaction is still present.

You will need to establish if you are allergic to tablets, etc. If a friend is already taking a preparation, ask nicely if they will give or sell a few tablets to start you off. Once you are happy that you are free of allergic reaction (and don't forget that it will not cause you to grow two heads even if you are) the treatment may commence.

Primary allergy

As I said earlier, primary allergy reveals itself by causing small mouth ulcers or blisters, a sore throat and itchy skin. These symptoms are all normally present, but may vary in degree. No degree of primary allergy is unduly distressing, but treatment should be discontinued if this reaction is experienced. A number of people ignore very mild symptoms and continue treatment, to find that after 7 days or thereabouts the reaction has disappeared and benefit is obtained. Other people ignore symptoms despite more than mild reaction, preferring the relatively minor discomfort of the allergy to the terrible pain of the primary ailment, and they have obviously derived sufficient benefit to make this a worthwhile proposition. The choice must be yours, however.

Secondary allergy

I used to call this 5-week allergy, not because it lasted for 5 weeks, but because it began to appear after this period of treatment. I didn't know why it happened initially, but the answers are now available. There are two basic causes:

1. Residual drugs

Certain synthetic drugs linger in the system for a considerable time. You may believe that you have been free of synthetic treatment for sufficient time to render the effect of such treatment to be ineffective as far as Feverfew is concerned, but unfortunately this is not always the case. Certain drugs cloak the initial or primary reaction for sufficient time to allow the Feverfew to build up until it is strong enough to break through. When this happens the primary allergy is released, but in a stronger form; mouth ulcers and blisters are more pronounced, the sore throat is more noticeable and swollen glands are introduced to the reaction. This form of allergic reaction may take up to a month to clear; it is not disabling, but you would certainly feel uncomfortable. Fortunately, it is so rare that only the immense amount of mail that I receive has given me the opportunity to spot it at all. A percentage of incidence would mean little because it is so rare.

2. Super efficiency

I couldn't think of anything else to call this subdivision, but it relates to those people who have derived the most benefit from Feverfew. These are the people who have not experienced migraine since Day 1, have felt considerable relief from arthritic pain within hours, or whose psoriasis has shown distinct improvement within a few days. The cause of the problem is build-up once again, but not because of allergy. It means quite simply that in the majority of cases these people are marvellously sympathetic to Feverfew and their requirements are tiny by comparison with the rest of us. It also implies that their systems are totally clear of related synthetics.

These are the people who must take care to reduce their intake of

Feverfew as soon as benefit is deemed to be reasonably established. This may be as early as two weeks, but should certainly be not later than four weeks if they wish to avoid the almost inevitable reaction. Such people should not be alarmed that they might lose the benefit bestowed by the herb. This will not happen. If everybody observed what I have said about reducing intake to minimal or even 0 once benefit is established, even the reaction would not be necessary.

Because the reaction in such cases is typical of allergy, it is possible to consider that such could be the cause. Since only you can tell, please, if you are one of the lucky people and there are many, please don't spoil the effect by continuing treatment when it is both unnecessary and undesirable for the reasons stated. You must have enough, I know, but do use common sense. This reaction is far more common than that from residual drugs because there are many people who fall into this category, and it is unlikely that they will ever require more than minimal top-up, if any. Once the original trauma has been cleared, only a new one will necessitate further treatment by Feverfew. This does not mean that if your response is slow but progressive you will not benefit equally. In this case both hare and tortoise can win.

Supplementary side-effects (allergy)

Apart from the two cases of palpitations mentioned in connection with concurrent treatment of Feverfew and high dosage blood pressure tablets, there have been very few adverse reports from the herb, and these have been of a mild and temporary nature. All have ceased within a few days of terminating Feverfew treatment.

Loss of appetite

This effect has now been reported by approximately 20 people. It is normally accompanied by loss of taste, and in all but one case it has been reported by leaf takers.

Dizziness

Dizziness has been reported by two people only, to whom I cannot offer good and sufficient reason, but it may well occur if you exceed the recommended dosage of good quality tablets. A single dosage of 150 mg is enough to make you dizzy, so if you are on an initial double dosage, do remember to split the dosage ½ morning and evening and don't forget to take it with food. This is important at any time, but particularly so with double dosage.

Diarrhea

No explanation is necessary with this one, but it is not too common an effect. At present it has reached double figures, but set against the number of testimonials I have received, one can hardly say that it has reached epidemic proportions. The longest time the problem has persisted after ceasing Feverfew treatment is seven days.

Increased appetite

This effect probably appears to be a funny thing to list with side-effects (allergy), but it might be a nuisance to anyone trying to maintain the appearance of a stick. Feverfew is peculiar in this respect. Because of its regulatory function, it may well cause your appetite to increase, because it thinks you are too thin for your own good. Fortunately, the two ladies who have experienced this effect are pleased about it, or I might have found myself in hot water.

Overefficiency

I know I have already mentioned this problem in the earlier section devoted to migraine, but it is the only case of its kind reported and therefore unique. It is not beyond the bounds of possibility that other people have experienced a similar reaction in cases of extreme sinus congestion. I would therefore greatly appreciate information from anyone similarly affected.

This section has been devoted entirely to allergic reaction, and the cases and types mentioned are all that have so far been reported.

Effects of concurrent dosage of Feverfew and other substances

Concurrent dosage with other substances is not a major problem with Feverfew, and up to press time there have been no terrible adverse reactions reported. By this I mean of the type that would occasion distress, like pain or vomiting. The reactions that mostly apply are twofold.

1. Synthetic drugs

Generally speaking, synthetic drugs retard the effectiveness of Feverfew to the extent that normal response times will probably not apply, so more time must be allowed for the herb to do its job.

Synthetics directed specifically at arthritis will probably cancel the effectiveness totally.

Drugs generally may have a cloaking effect on allergy to the extent discussed in the allergy section. Drugs normally prescribed in connection with migraine and arthritis are for the most part, painkillers only. Few aspire to a cure, so you have little to lose by speaking to your doctor about Feverfew. Logically it is merely an extension of treatment, and while it may not offer a cure in all cases, it does offer pain relief without side-effects and many other benefits as described in the testimonials.

You may not have sufficient confidence in Feverfew to do without painkillers for a few days, though many have done so and been rewarded for their faith. If you do find it necessary to take painkillers during the initial stages of treatment, stick to over-the-counter types, for these have no appreciable retarding effect. A double dosage of Feverfew normally takes care of the pain problem encountered during the first few days.

2. Alcohol

There are many people who are only too ready to tell you that alcohol has no effect on Feverfew. They are wrong. Some of these people are herbalists, even homeopathic doctors. They are doing the herb a great disservice, insofar as alcohol affects Feverfew in the vast majority of cases. I am not attempting to cover my back by saying "the vast majority" because I am well aware that some people may benefit, even though they take alcohol and Feverfew concurrently. Nevertheless I stand by what I have said.

The important thing to realize is that you will never know precisely how much benefit you may derive unless you take the herb without the alcohol. Taking both together does not make you sick or ill, so there are no obvious signs that you are receiving short change from the herb. Is there any form or minimum quantity of alcohol that will not have adverse effect? The answer is no to both; wine to whisky, millilitres to hogsheads, *NO*. Be fair, you will be only too ready to say that you have not received benefit when you have combined the two, as some people have already done. In the end they have had to admit that they have not appreciated that a social drink is still alcohol, whatever the reason. I am not a teetotaller by any means, so don't go away with the impression that I am using a back door on behalf of the Temperance Society.

First, establish what the herb has to offer and then you can go back to your booze if you must, but I warn you that the odds are long against your receiving benefit at all, let alone maximum benefit. If you have given the herb a fair trial in this respect and then you do take a drink, the chances are that the pain will return immediately. The choice is then yours; nobody can make it for you.

If you need a little encouragement, I can tell you of a gentleman from a seaside town who had become a controlled alcoholic. He tried Feverfew and naturally received little or no benefit, but he was aware of what I had to say about alcohol and he had this choice to make. It must have been terrible for him but he gave up his drink to take the herb. I was more pleased than I can say when he received his reward in freedom from pain.

The herb is very forgiving and if you stray from the path, the full benefit normally returns within 48 hours of resuming treatment, provided you then abstain from alcohol.

Dosage

On the odd occasions over the years that letters have been printed relative to the benefits of Feverfew, I have been surprised at that variation of dosage suggested. The fact that only Feverfew is mentioned rather than a specific variety is not relevant to this section except for the fact that you might consume acres of Golden Feverfew in connection with arthritis or psoriasais without gaining an ounce of benefit. So once again I stress that I concern myself solely with *Tanacetum parthenium* (Wild Feverfew) of a high quality, and dosages recommended are given on that same understanding.

It must also be understood that when I refer to tablets or other commercial preparations, I am thinking only of good quality products with a high level of activity. However, over the years I have arrived at an optimum dosage, and as optimum dosages have a habit of doing, it works quite well, being flexible over the initial 10-14 days because of individual requirements.

You have read about the full effects of allergic reaction, and as a new starter you must have regard to this possible effect. If you are starting with fresh leaf, you will encounter the highest possible chance of hitting the allergy, because at 7% it has the highest incidence of any form of

Feverfew. You will then need to measure, because the optimum daily dosage is 2 × 2½-inch leaves, approximately 125 mg dried herb.

I assume that you have already been tested for allergy. If not, I suggest that you do so. Initial dosage is important, and you will have to choose which dosage applies to you.

Arthritis and migraine

Arthritis (at onset stage), migraine (at monthly intervals or more), stress (in early stages, i.e., not requiring tranquilizers), insomnia

All of the above should respond adequately to daily dosage of 125 mg. Of course this may be either in tablet form or fresh leaf. In the case of insomnia the Feverfew should be taken at night. A particularly effective way of making up a sleeping potion is to take two leaves, brew them as tea, and leave until cool enough to drink.

Arthritis (in developed stage with heavy pain, stiff limbs, etc., sore and swollen joints), migraine (severe at less than monthly intervals), stress (requiring regular tranquilizers), spondylitus

At this stage in developed ailments, double dosage is advisable for an initial period of 10-14 days. If you find that relief is rapid, reduce the dosage to 125 mg as soon as you feel confident, because you may be one of the people mentioned in the allergy section whose metabolic reaction is swift and favourable, but who may achieve rapid build-up and allergic reaction as a consequence if dosage is not reduced.

Menopause, P.M.T.

To treat menopause and premenstrual tension only single dosage is required. Feverfew must be taken as a course until you derive benefit and feel confident that you can reduce to top-up only and finally to cessation of treatment. Don't be afraid to experiment with dosage; you will not lose what you have gained.

Please observe the following:

1. Take Feverfew with food whenever possible.
2. Do not chew raw leaves. Yes sir, I know *you* can, *but*. . . .!

3. With double dosage take 125 mg night and morning.
4. Do not take Feverfew with high dosage blood pressure tablets.
5. Do not take alcohol during the initial treatment period.
6. Do experiment to reduce dosage as soon as you feel confident. It is not necessary to continue full dosage forevermore. Once you have achieved a reasonable stage, the herb will continue to work for you. Just like a microwave oven, the effect will continue after the power supply has been cut off.

The curative effect of Feverfew does not die off simply because you have chosen to discontinue treatment. If you read the testimonials carefully, you will discover periods of relief ranging from months to years during which relief has been maintained without further treatment.

Experiment to see how long you can go without treatment once benefit is established; you could be in for a big surprise. Even if the pain does begin to return, it will only be gradual, giving you ample time to top-up a bit sharpish.

Psoriasis

I have kept this section apart because psoriasis cannot comfortably be mixed with either of the other two sections. Like the other ailments, relief may be obtained in a few days, but degree of coverage requires different dosages if you wish to consolidate benefit within a reasonable time. In the case of arthritis and migraine much of the dosage is absorbed as a painkiller, so only light coverage will respond quickly to single dosage in most cases. If coverage is dense and extensive, it will probably be necessary to take double dosage for up to three months. So do remember what I have said about the reaction due to build-up, and be prepared to reduce to a single dosage as soon as benefit begins to make itself felt.

Efficacy of different preparations

During my early years of research I confined myself solely to the study of the efficacy of fresh leaf and its attendant allergy ratio, but I had searched diligently throughout the U.K. and abroad for dried Feverfew or tablets. I searched because I reasoned that there could well be a difference between the allergy ratios, but in the end my first "patient" beat me to the draw. Whilst on holiday in South Wales he accompanied a fellow holidaymaker to a health food shop to buy Feverfew tablets; yes, as easily as that. His companion had used them for some time with considerable relief.

This was a great stride forward, and I made haste to buy some for my wife. Her reaction was exactly the same, so once again I was deeply disappointed in this respect. I began to tell people about the tablets, and the small firm that produced them quickly sold out. This was most unfortunate, as there could be no more until the following year, or so I thought, but the lady owner was totally dedicated to the cause of Feverfew, and she managed to buy in from abroad. Only small quantities of genuine herb were available, but she managed to supply my "patients" by mail order, although there was not sufficient herb to put tablets into shops.

Since that time, of course, the market has been flooded with Feverfew preparations of various types, having various levels of activity. I have been fortunate in having been advised of the results of trials directed specifically at levels of activity in products bought over the counter. It is absolutely astounding how much different preparations vary, with levels of activity ranging between 0 and 100, the yardstick being fresh leaf.

There was no luck involved in settling on the tablet of my choice because I had the benefit of testimonials to guide me. Not only did I receive information relative to the tablets I recommended on the basis of local results, but I was also informed of the negative results encountered in others. A recognizable pattern emerged, and as the variety of preparations grew so did the league table of results.

Herbal tablets

I may appear to be partisan in my preference for *herbal tablets*, but I am in fact directed by the sheer weight of testimonials in this direction. I have kept an open mind and have given every opportunity for other types of preparations to establish themselves. I feel that this cannot simply be coincidence, but I am mindful of the fact that if anybody has asked my opinion, I have given it without fear or favour. One recommendation for herbal tablets has already been withdrawn because of falling standards. Since I do not own shares in any laboratory, I can speak simply on the basis of results.

Another manufacturer was advised, not only about a faulty batch, but also about a faulty counting machine, all on the basis of information gleaned from correspondence, of which I have no shortage whatsoever. The machine was overhauled and a reason sought for the substandard batch. When this problem came to light, it was easily rectified and the standard has remained high ever since. Had it not been so, there would have been another recommendation stricken from the list, but this particular tablet is now the yardstick by which other are judged. The person who gave me this information had has an impeccable pedigree and no commercial affiliations whatsoever, but he rates this tablet very highly by comparison with any other commercial product in terms of level in activity. There can be no higher praise as far as I am concerned. My hope for the future is that the level will be maintained.

This standard has set a very high target for other manufacturers to aim at, and as the league table shows, there is none within 50% of its level, but there are many below even the 50% level, even 0, and there can be no excuse for this. I appreciate that some manufacturers have fallen short through ignorance, but my work has always been freely available to all. It is possible, to ruin a batch simply by cutting the correct herb at the wrong time, so you can imagine part of the problem. The herb is as precious as the finest grapes in this respect, but while you may decide that a wine is worth buying by the various methods adopted by connoisseurs, you can't do this with Feverfew. Only lack of results will tell you if you have been sold a dud or not.

What finally determines the quality of the tablet? Naturally it must be guaranteed *Tanacetum parthenium,* and unfortunately this is not always the case. This does not mean that the manufacturer is being dishonest, and you do have the benefit of the Trades Descriptions Act in this respect. Obviously, however, it is not an offence simply to put the name Feverfew on the packet if it contains Feverfew of whichever variety. No license has yet been granted for Feverfew in respect to arthritis, migraine and psoriasis, so manufacturers may not specify the ailment for which the herb is being sold. It is sold as a "food supplement."

I have seen both sides of the coin, for I have been asked if I could locate supplies for good quality herb, and I have been asked if I would like to buy good quality herb. Since I am not commercially involved with any manufacturer or grower, and I do not charge fees for any help I am able to give, I feel that I have the right to request fullest details of the herb before I complete a transfer between interested parties. I believe that if anyone has the confidence in my judgment it should not be abused. For this reason, I will not accept recommendations for the herb unless it is accompanied by a certificate of authenticity in the first place, and it must then be confirmed by laboratory tests. You would be surprised how often a vendor loses interest when I mention certificates and laboratory tests.

One drawback with tablets in the U.K. at present is the use of bone phosphate as the primary filler: this has a tendency to restrict the market somewhat in connection with certain religious groups or vegetarians. Since I have brought this matter to their attention, some manufacturers in this country have begun the process of changing over to mineral fillers. I cannot see that this will have an adverse effect on tablets as far as level of activity is concerned, but the effect of the filler, though theoretically unlikely to affect anybody adversely, has yet to be seen. It may be necessary to continue the bone phosphate for certain groups.

Do watch what you are buying in the tablet line. Most of the reputable manufacturers are now specifying *Tanacetum parthenium* as the herb content, but it is still possible to find combination names using those alternative names mentioned at the beginning of the book. If the package merely states Feverfew, be careful. I do not at present know of any such tablets that rate even a reasonable level of activity.

Capsules

It was not until 1984 that capsules began to appear in quantity in the Feverfew market place. I was aware of only one firm that produced capsules, and these were to special order only, handfilled by the proprietor of a small firm in South Wales for people who could not take tablets or were unwilling for whatever reason to consume the filler/binder. They are more acceptable outside the United Kingdom which appears to have a preference for tablets that is not shared outside these sunny shores. Be that as it may, if they contain the correct herb in the optimum dosage range, they are perfectly acceptable and are certainly more adaptable than tablets.

Because capsules have only been on the market a short while, it has not been possible for me to assess their value in relative terms. Up to press the number of testimonials that has mentioned them is small, and it is on these that I must base my assessment. Dosage restrictions still apply, however.

General medical opinion

You have read various comments regarding the attitude of medical practitioners. I will now try to show both sides of the coin in a relatively short section devoted specifically to this subject.

'I was so impressed that I had to tell my doctor. . . . he was quite interested.' Testimonial 273.

'. . . . but a few weeks ago I met a lady who for years had suffered from migraine. She went to a migraine clinic and Feverfew is what they told her to take. Apparently she is no longer a migraine sufferer.'
Estimonial 275.

'It may be of interest to know that I mentioned this to a Harley Street consultant and he was not in the slightest bit surprised at the beneficial effects of Feverfew. I should add that Feverfew was not a placebo as I didn't expect it to work.'
Testimonial 286.

'I further requested my doctor to stop the xxxxxx tablets as I was taking Feverfew and he obliged.'
Testimonial 307.

'When I told my doctor he just laughed, said I was naive and if it was so good why hadn't the big drug companies manufactured it.' Testimonial 318.

'As a matter of interest the friend who had found Feverfew helpful was phoned by the migraine clinic. The lady said "We haven't heard from you lately" and my friend replied "I've been taking Feverfew". The lady said "I know Feverfew, carry on with it." Testimonial 28.

'We urged her to try Feverfew. She took our advice and told her doctor. We were all agreeably surprised when he said he would give her Feverfew tablets.'
Testimonial 117.

'I have taken Feverfew for three months with excellent results . . . I am not on any drugs, and my doctor is in favour of my taking Feverfew.' Testimonial 223.

Degree of relief

How does one assess the degree of relief that has been obtained by treatment with Feverfew? It is entirely relative, and what may appear miraculous to one person may be accepted as only reasonable by another.

A person gaining relief from twice yearly migraine will not be as impressed as someone who has been relieved of thrice weekly migraine. Someone who is experiencing the onset of arthritis will never comprehend the satisfaction of a person who has given up a walking frame or even a wheelchair. One could go on like this, but I think the point is made.

I have received letters from people who have said that they had reached the stage of believing that Feverfew had done little for them so they had returned to the social world and alcohol. They found that the herb had in fact done a fair bit of work, as was shown when alcohol killed the beneficial effect. In the main these people had only taken the herb for a short while, and benefit was not fully established.

What are you expecting from the herb? Don't aim for a miracle and be disappointed. Once you have read the testimonials you will have gained a very good idea of what you may expect, and do be assured that there is no reason why you should not receive adequate benefit if you use a bit of common sense. You may not know if you are on foot or horseback at present because of pain and distress, but tomorrow is another day. It could be a Feverfew day, and the world might quickly take on a fresh perspective.

One section of Feverfewites is devoted to those who have been able to return to former sporting glory, golf most prominently but also mentioned are bowls and badminton. So far nobody has expressed a desire to return to *Sumo* wrestling; this I can understand having tried it once in Singapore. They couldn't find a uniform small enough for me.

Just remember that if you couldn't run a mile in 4 minutes pre-Feverfew, it is not likely that you will be able to do it post-Feverfew. No matter how good you feel, I think you should take a hard look at yourself before deciding on a return to knitting or the Admiral's Cup.

What does the future hold?

A good question this is, and I am glad you asked. At present trials are being conducted into the efficacy of Feverfew in connection with arthritis, migraine and psoriasis in the United Kingdom and abroad. Thanks to the generosity of a manufacturer I have been able to supply active and placebo tablets to two universities which are conducting such trials. The manufacturer does not know where his tablets have gone, and the universities don't know where they have come from. At this stage of the game it is better that way.

I am hopeful that with the assistance of a third university, further trials will soon commence in connection with psoriasis; there is no point in further delay. There have been enquiries for information from various centres in this connection but nothing concrete so far with regard to trials. Someone is missing a golden opportunity.

I shall continue with my research for I really have no option. Until people stop writing to me—God forbid—I shall carry on. Because of what I have already in the pipeline, and that which will undoubtedly come to light through testimonials yet to come, I have no doubt that 1986 will see more exciting news from Feverfew, and it *will* be in the van of a herbal renaissance.

Until I have more proof concerning these latest developments I shall say no more, but evidence relative to psoriasis was slow to begin rolling in. Once it started, however, it was a positive indication that it was not simply a placebo effect in the odd case or two. The herb has much more to offer, but I certainly do not wish to raise false hopes. For this reason I shall search diligently for more proof until I am satisfied and then you too will know.

How do I grow Feverfew?

There is very little that can be said in this respect, for as many gardeners will tell you, the plant self-sets profusely. It can be difficult to start from seed; in any event a plant grown from seed is not going to be readily available for medicinal purposes until it is two years old. Better by far is it to purchase a plant, stick it in a spot in the garden in semi-shade and you will have the benefit not only of a beautifully decorative plant, but a medicine chest as well.

At present seeds are quite scarce, but they are obtainable. Do ensure that the correct variety is obtained; I have given you the alternatives at the beginning of the book, so if you have forgotten them, you will have to start reading through again.

I have seen some weird and wonderful plants being offered as Feverfew, so I do urge you to buy from reputable growers. The wrong variety may be sold in ignorance, but that will not help you in 12 months' time when you come to use it and find that you have bought another variety of Feverfew.

Please do accept my word for it that a mature Feverfew plant does not like plant pots. More have died in these than outside in a severe winter.

All my research plants have survived the winter and are perking up beautifully. From the beginning of April they will begin to shoot up.

I can't sell you seeds or plants, for as I have said so many times before, I have only research stock. A great number of specimens are sent to me for identification, but very few arrive in a recognizable state; usually they are simply slime. They are adequate facilities in most areas where the herb may be identified, and I urge you to try these first, avoiding disappointment when I have to write to tell you that the specimen was unrecognizable.

Where can I buy Feverfew preparation?

Just about every health food shop and drugstore stocks Feverfew of one type or another. The range of dosage is quite baffling, some being below what I consider to be the optimum and others well above. The range of levels of activity within these products is amazing and is directly responsible for the variation in results, or lack of same.

Short of producing a list of all products with recommendations I can only advise that if you have any doubt with regard to any product, write to Kathy Turner, 86 Holly Avenue, Breaston, Derby DE73BR. Her company has a product that has been produced to a specification built upon hundreds of testimonials and has produced superb results. Do bear in mind that I am not saying that other products will not do the same, but I am extremely jealous of the reputation of the herb, and I intensely dislike receiving letters telling me that the herb does not work, when after a course of a proven product, these same people gain wonderful benefit. The damage has already been done. There is no way that these people will go back and cancel what they have already said to damn the name of the herb, and me too if it comes to that.

Feverfew works if you give it a chance.

A high-quality tablet, using the precise strain of Feverfew recommended, was developed and is manufactured by ABCO Laboratories, of Concord, California, in a unique freeze-dry-Lyophilized-process. It is available at health food stores and pharmacies.

The efficacy of herbal preparations is determined by several critical factors, including the viability and purity of the seeds, environmental conditions, timing the harvest drying of the herbs, extraction of the active ingredients and incorporated into the finished product. Every batch must meet these stringent conditions to insure a product of standardized potency.

Lyphoherb is an exclusive process which insures that all of these conditions are met before its seal of approval appears on the finished products. The following criteria apply to all Lyphoherb products:

1. VIABILITY AND PURITY OF THE SEEDS

Seeds are selected by plant geneticists to insure that only the correct subspecies of a particular herb are used. The seeds are tested for viability prior to planting.

2. ENVIRONMENTAL CONDITIONS

The optimal growing conditions are determined beforehand by a consulting plant physiologist. The proper soil conditions, temperature, moisture, sunlight and length of the growing season are supervised by scientifically trained agronomists. Each particular species of herb is subject to a different environmental protocol. This is why it is necessary to cultivate different herbs in different parts of the country and thus insure an herbal product of the highest quality.

3. TIMING OF THE HARVEST

No herb is harvested before its time. In some cases, the herb must be harvested before the flower blooms. In other cases, depending on the herb, it should be harvested prior to seeding.

4. DRYING OF THE HERBS

Lyphoherb protects the active constituents of the herbs during drying and manufacturing. It stands for true lyophilization, otherwise known as freeze-drying. According to reproducible chromotography studies, freeze-drying was shown to produce a far superior product to herbs dried by other methods (i.e., sun-dried, air-dried). The active alkaloids, volatile oils and colors are retained to insure that these critical components of the natural plant are not denatured during manufacturing.

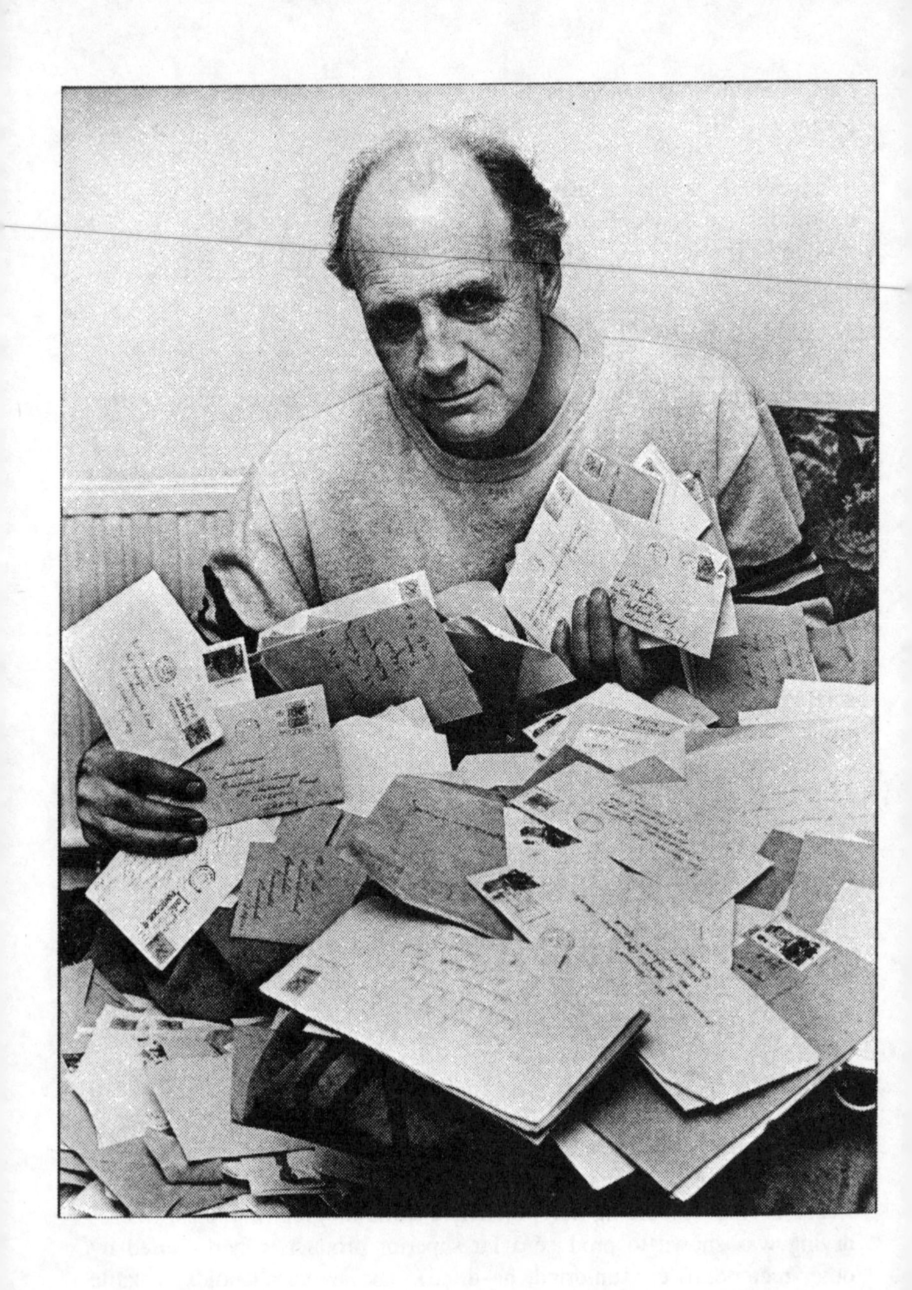

Testimonials
(affidavits)

The testimonials in this section are a sample taken from those sent to me between July 1984 and January 1985. They are in edited form because many of them are 2-3 pages and some as long as 8 pages.

Each in its own way forms part of the Feverfew story as I see it, and if you study them closely you will find much of interest. I feel that there cannot be one family that cannot identify with a number of them; even if you are not personally affected by any of the ailments mentioned, I am sure that at least one member of your family will be able so to identify.

The originals of all testimonials are retained for purposes of validation. Application by official bodies for a sight of these documents should be made to the author at 80, Holbrook Road, Alvaston, Derby DE2 0DF, England.

It is a simple matter to decide which of the testimonials are of value to research, and I ask you most sincerely to examine your own case in depth and then write to me, giving your own experience. There is yet much to be learned about this herb, and I stress that I would appreciate *details* of all experiences, good, bad or indifferent. Tell me if you are taking drugs at the same time and what they are, and if you have recently completed a course of synthetics.

You can see what Feverfew has done for the people whose testimonials are included, but please bear in mind that the number is small by comparison with the whole. There is immense interest in Feverfew, and you can play your part in unfolding the story to the benefit of thousands, nay millions of sufferers.

Thank you in advance for your cooperation. Letters should be addressed to the International Feverfew Appreciation Society at the above address. But if you require an answer, please do remember that since I finance my own research, a stamped, self-addressed envelope would be appreciated.

'Dear Ken Hancock,
I am beside myself with joy; but before I get too carried away let me tell you, in the shortest way possible.
Today is the 8th day taking Feverfew. Before that my doctor had given me endless drugs to no avail, one being xxxxxx that made me very ill after just one pill, seven people died taking these things. A lot of people persist in taking anything a doctor prescribes, despite the bad reaction;

they are too afraid to refuse them, not having the sense to realize drug companies are experimenting, and where else but through doctors and the trusting public.
For the past two years the use of my legs became a torture, so bad in fact only on rare days during the past year I've been able to walk. I'd shuffle, have to stop, pain tearing at me, feeling like a fool standing there unable to move, tears streaming down my face. Then I read a tiny piece of information about you. I do not believe it, *BUT* I was so depressed and so desperate I'd try anything, because believe me, if I was to wind up in a wheel chair a large dose of sleeping pills would be the only way out. When I give you my background you will understand that I'm no coward. After the second day I felt different; I put it down to wishful thinking. Day 4 I got on a bus, went shopping for three hours. I did not stop or sit down, only twice, five minutes there and back to xxxxxx xxxx xxxxxxx. I had an ache in my legs that's all. I still refused to believe. Day 7. Ran around non-stop for 5 hours, I went mad with happiness; blessed you and your pretty little flowers, talked to everyone, had two people get up there and then to buy Feverfew. There are no words, no action, no gift that would be good enough to thank you.'

1

(In view of the nature of this testimonial and the identity of the person concerned, I have taken steps to check its authenticity. It is genuine and before editing it ran into 8 pages. Author)

'I am overweight and 62 . . . . most of the women in my family suffer from a general stiffness . . . . and we all have enlarged finger joints and toe joints to some degree, and suffer pain.
I went to my doctor 10 years ago and she told me I had osteoarthritis. . . . "something one has to learn to live with." Last summer, June '83 I developed a terrible pain under my right heel, I was in agony. . . . I really got quite frightened at the thought of being crippled, and became so depressed. At this time too I heard that the drug I had been taking for 10 years had been withdrawn. I remember seeing that Feverfew was good for arthritis, and had some in the garden.
Within a month all the pain had gone and I stopped taking the Feverfew. In May of this year a similar pain developed in the other foot and I started taking the Feverfew again. After I had stripped the plant I went onto tablets. The pain is completely gone. I show your leaflet to every sufferer I meet, and shall always sing the praises of Feverfew.'

2

'It is 7 months since I started taking Feverfew, and as well as relief from arthritis, my migraine is almost a thing of the past. I can really put it down to nothing but Feverfew.'

7

'. . . . after suffering for many years from severe attacks of migraine. The relief was indescribable when my attacks became less frequent, and it is now two years since I had an attack.'

8

'I am over 60 years of age, have taken "your" Feverfew tablets for just over 6 weeks and can honestly say they do me good. My headaches are not quite as severe, arthritis not so painful, I am sleeping better and feel brighter (I find myself bursting into song occasionally). Constipation is not such a problem as it was. . . .'

9

'. . . .I couldn't believe it when I walked into town and back the other day with no pain. It was wonderful, my feet had wings.'

10

'My doctor only prescribed painkillers for arthritis in the hips which was crippling me to the extent that I had to go up and down stairs one step at a time. I can now put equal weight on both legs and walk normally.'

18

'I have been taking tablets daily since I read your article in the Daily Mail, and I am amazed at the relief of pain.'

21

'I have had wonderful relief from migraine since taking Feverfew, and my husband has now started to eat leaves in the hope that he will get relief from painful arthritis in his knees.'

25

'Thank you for telling me about Feverfew. I have been taking it, and have not had a migraine since. I got migraine with my period.'

27

'When you first wrote to the Daily Mail regarding Feverfew I told a friend who suffered from migraine about it. I somehow thought it had not been heeded. However four months later this friend said ''Thank you for telling me about Feverfew, it has helped.''
I have been interested in the correspondence, especially the letter from the gentleman who said that he had given it to two arthritic Labradors and was amazed at the result.
As a matter of interest the friend who has found Feverfew helpful was phoned by the migraine clinic. The lady said ''We haven't heard from you lately,'' and my friend said ''I've been taking Feverfew.'' The lady said ''I know Feverfew, carry on with it.'' '

28

'In 1969 I began taking the contraceptive pill and within 6 months I had my first migraine attack. . . . I had not heard of migraine so I thought I was suffering from a 24-hour bug. I began to get my bug more frequently. . . . I read a newspaper article about migraine and realized what I was suffering from.
The article said that women on the pill frequently have migraine whereas they hadn't before taking it. I changed to the lowest dosage pill but the migraine continued unabated, so I changed my method of contraception. I took no more pills, but was dismayed to discover that the migraines was here to stay. I tried various remedies from the chemist without effect; anitmigraine tablets make me vomit.
Happily my father read about Feverfew versus migraine . . . migraine is now gone I am pleased to say. I ate two leaves every day at one time, but I haven't had any regularly since migraine finished a year ago. Whilst gardening I occasionally eat a leaf or two.'

31

'I have derived great benefit from taking this herb for 15 months. My migraines have lessened, and when I have one it is bearable. The pain from arthritis is now non-existent. It is a remarkable herb.'

32

'I must have been one of the 5000 correspondents who wrote to you after reading your letters in the Daily Mail last year. At that time my West Highland Terrier had developed arthritis in one back leg and was pretty miserable. I took her to the vet, who gave her the inevitable injection and pills with no good result. So I wrote away for Feverfew tablets, and

within a week or so there was a decided ''lightening of the spirit'' as you say, and within a few weeks she was chasing the squirrels and was able to jump onto my bed again (worse luck), which she had been unable to do when she had developed arthritis
I have passed your letter on to a number of people; the only trouble is that they take such a long time to bring it back.'

42

'For 6 years I have suffered arthritis of the knee . . . but about 3 weeks ago I was given some tablets to try. What can I say? My knee is no longer stiff, and I can walk without rolling and limping. I feel 99% better.'

43

'I have arthritis in both feet and my neck, and started taking Feverfew merely in the hope of delaying the worsening symptoms. I did not wish to risk strong drugs with side-effects probably worse than my symptoms. Five years ago I also went deaf and have used a hearing aid for the last few months. This last week my hearing has begun to improve, and it had not occurred to me that it could be the arthritis in my neck. *I am not imagining* my improved hearing.'

45

'My daughter has found Feverfew to be the real answer (the only answer) to many years of bad migraine. She is a staff nurse.'

46

'I have been taking 2 leaves of Feverfew in a sandwich daily for the past 15 months for migraine. I might add that they were very bad migraines, as many as 2-4 in a month, putting me out of action for 1 or even 2 days at a time. I am now aged 57 and suffered from them all my life; only wish I had known about it years ago, especially when my children were young. I noticed a marked improvement after 4 months of taking it and now the migraines have completely gone.'

52

'I have been taking Feverfew tablets for 3 weeks and must say how well they are, I have so much less pain. I have been suffering from arthritis for 40 years, I am 81. Now after just 3 weeks can't explain how much easier it is for me, getting more rest, and also getting around better in such a short time after taking so many pills and painkillers. Thank you for making it possible for me to get so much relief.'

59

'. . . . completely abolished the menopausal curse—hot flushes.'

60

'I am also convinced that Feverfew has had a considerable relief to the amount of early morning cramp (5 a.m.-6 a.m.) which has bothered me most of my life.'

63

'I too can now walk with greater ease (osteoarthritis), and nearly all the swelling is gone, but what really does amaze me is that the hard lumps on the joints of my ankles have almost gone.'

65

'Although I have Feverfew in my garden I cannot take it in its natural form. The tablets I have found to be most effective in the control of psoriasis. I have suffered from this in all parts of the body and scalp for 59 years.'

66

'My husband has been using some for several months, and has had tremendous relief from his arthritis. I would appreciate your broadsheet to send to my sister in Canada.'

73

'I have been taking Feverfew for a week now, as I have arthritis in my legs, and I have found much benefit from it. Just as I am writing this letter I feel no pain at all which is really marvellous. I wish I'd heard about it before as I was getting crippled.'

79

'You started me on the Feverfew trail about 2 years ago when I was in pain with my hip, since then I have been free from pain.'

82

'I have a damaged spine (3 twisted vertebrae in the center of my back) and arthritis had set in from the neck to the bottom of my spine. For quite a few years I have been in constant pain and the stiffness was getting very inconvenient. The doctors only help was to offer painkillers, which I was going to stay clear of as along as possible. . . . Feverfew has given me a new lease on life. I can't tell you how grateful I am to be almost free from stiffness and to have little or no pain, and to be able to sleep at night. Thank you very much for sending them to two of my friends who are also benefiting from them.'

94

'I have suffered with ankylosing spondylitis for 3 years (since 18), and I started taking Feverfew 2 months ago after having to take steroids to get me through my wedding day. It is great to find something that gives the relief without side-effects.'

96

'I have found a Health shop selling the tablets, and I am definitely not getting migraine after suffering it for some years. I did not know about migraine until I had a gall bladder operation (removal) 8 years ago; since then I have had a bad time.'

97

'I started taking Feverfew last December, '83. I know how much good it has done me. I thought it was about time I came off tablets. If I may be bold enough to ask you for three leaflets, as I want to send one to the U.S.A., another to Canada.'

101

'Previously I took xxxxxx tablets prescribed by my doctor, but they had very severe side-effects, so I stopped taking them and started with Feverfew having read your article in the Trader.
They proved very beneficial; gradually my legs which had been very stiff and painful became completely free of arthritis. I have every confidence in the Feverfew tablets and would recommend them to anyone with arthritis.'

103

'Suffering great pain in my right knee I went to the doctor. His verdict was "Arthritis at your age (60), it won't cripple you. No cure, just give you painkillers." I didn't take them and I didn't go back. At the end of September, I saw a paragraph in a paper about Feverfew for arthritis, so I sent to you for a month supply which I received and started taking the first week in September. At that time I could not put my leg out straight or bend it very far up, and could not kneel and was limping badly never without severe pain. Since starting the tablets relief started within days and has increased every day since . . . Yesterday and today I have walked up over the snow-covered hills and fields behind my house, yesterday for 1 hour 40 minutes, today for 1 hour 20 minutes, non-stop both times, covering over three miles . . . What a wonderful feeling after 3 years of pain.'

104

'' . . . . As I've noticed that they are helping with my psoriasis which has been persistent for years.'

105

'For the past 4 weeks I have been taking your Feverfew pills for my arthritis and have found them a big success. For 18 years I have been a sufferer, and thanks to Feverfew I no longer feel any pain.'

114

'I have a catalogue of physical problems, and most things for arthritis don't suit diverticulitis. Have tried Feverfew for one week and found hands were so much better.'

116

'In the early 1970s I was examined and told rather brutally ''You have arthritis in the neck, spine, hips, knees and hands. It is an incurable disease, you will probably be crippled, but will have to learn to live with it.''

I was then in my early 50s and had to give up a good job, and was practically confined to the house for the next 2 years.

I am convinced that if I had continued to take all the drugs offered by the medical profession I would not be alive today. For instance I was given xxxxxx and recommended to take 12 daily, before it was discovered that 8 daily could be fatal. I was also given xxxxxxxx which fortunately I did not take.

It may surprise you to know that I have just returned from a brisk mile walk over the mountain. Apart from the odd twinge I lived a normal life. My friend, an elderly lady who lives in the Isle of Man had derived great

benefit from Feverfew for her rheumatism. She pours boiling water on the leaves and soaks a bandage in the liquid . . .
. . . . about his wife who suffered from migraine. We urged her to try Feverfew. She took our advice and told her doctor. We were all agreeably surprised when he said that he would give her Feverfew tablets. She hasn't had an attack for over two months now.'

117

'I have been eating Feverfew for the least 12 months, with astounding results re: migraine.'

118

'Please send me your revised broadsheet in connection with Feverfew. Some of my patients have mentioned it as being of great benefit, and I feel sure that others could be interested.'

122

'. . . . and I can again knit and sew for hours on end, even fine sewing which was previously extremely painful and I could only do for very short periods.'

125

'This really is an S.O.S. I have been using Feverfew tablets for 10 days on the recommendation of a friend, and find them beneficial. I would like to continue treatment, *BUT* I am due to return to New Zealand on Sept. 12th. I enclose cash for a 3 month supply, also please supply details of an agent in New Zealand.'

126

'I have paraplegia caused by damage to the motor nerves due to spondylosis and displacement of 4 bones in the neck. I have been like this for 16 years. For the last six months I have taken *only* Feverfew, which I have obtained from Jack and Kathy Turner, and have had considerable relief from pain with no side-effects.'

128

'. . . . and felt like a guinea pig. I feel that I have tried most of the drugs on the market, many of which had awful side-effects and don't work. The only one that I felt had any effect without nausea was xxxx which of course has now been withdrawn. I turned to Feverfew after reading a letter in the Daily Mail, but didn't really believe it would work. Well, so far it has, fingers crossed. (ankylosing spondylitus).'

132

'I have suffered with arthritis of the neck, knee joints and hands for about three years now, and have tried all the remedies that have been told me, and that I have read about, with no success. If I wanted to look around I had to turn my whole body around, and my knees were so swollen, making it difficult to walk, as were my hands. But since taking Feverfew I can turn my head in any direction. Now the swelling on my knee joints has gone, so have the swellings on my hands. Apart from slight stiffness of the neck muscles. I am back to my old self. I also suffered from migraine headaches. These too have gone, a thing I have not known for years. I cannot find words enough to thank you."

136

'Thank you for your leaflet on Feverfew. As a result I am taking the tablets mainly to help with my arthritis. You will be interested in my comments about the tablets I expect.

1. My aches and pains from arthritis have improved. I have only taken the tablets for 10 days.
2. Trouble with migraine has vanished.
3. Menopausal problems have greatly improved.'

137

'. . . . my husband and I have both had good results, both sufferers of arthritis. . . . He has had movement in his wrist after taking Feverfew, as only treatment from the hospital could do, but that was short-lived after treatment.
I have for some years had my vision marred (not to blindness), but by a kind of black net before my eyes which seemed to dull the vision. I had examinations at xxxxxxx (very extensive) at the beginning but was just told it was not serious, but was not given any reason. I also have arthritis in my neck. . . . this was not so bad when taking the leaves, also I woke one morning to find that my sight was much brighter. I am looking forward to taking the leaves or tablets again . . . at the moment I have that faint blur back. I can remember my mother going to xxxxxxx in her later years and they told her it was nothing. . . . she had trouble, her eyes got very sore and she herself maintained it was arthritis . . . Our

daughter also has found relief taking the tablets she sent to Derby for, she suffered with migraine.'

154

'I just had to write and tell you what a wonderful tablet Feverfew is. My mum (95) spent days in bed because she couldn't walk with arthritis in her hip and leg. She has been taking the tablet now for 3 weeks and can walk on her own with her stick. I have also got some for my sister and a friend on my way into town.'
(Two days after receiving the above letter I was informed by telephone that 'mum' was now climbing stairs without assistance. Author)

157

'I sent for Feverfew 4 weeks ago and sir, I cannot say how grateful I am that I sent for them. I am 82, have had osteoarthritis for over 19 years, have a plastic shoulder, one hand 17 stitches because it almost closed up, now I was going to have one on my left one, but since taking one month supply of Feverfew my hand is straightened so I cancelled my op. I have suffered so much pain in my left knee, and was told at xxxx Hospital no use going unless I was in dire distress, they could do no more for me. . . . 15 very wide steps outside my flat . . . I can now do each step in one go . . . since Feverfew no pain in my knee. I thank God every day for the relief.'

164

'The results are fantastic, after 20 years of suffering and so crippled I could barely walk, with advanced arthritis of both knees and feet. I am very grateful for the help I am getting from Feverfew.'

167

'I have been for 20 years a psoriasis sufferer. Doctors, Specialists, Faith healers, Hypnosis, all have failed, but after 1 week of Feverfew the irritation has gone and now the patches have diminished, the soreness gone and the discoloration fading.
To say I am delighted is to put it mildly, so I am starting my sister and a friend on them, to see if it will work for them.'

168

'I would like to thank you for sending me your information on Feverfew at the end of July. . . . and must say that I am truly amazed at the

painrelieving powers of Feverfew, which I have been taking now for just over two months.
I am 68 years of age and have had pain in hips, thighs, back and knees for some years. Then just before last Xmas I had an acute attack of sciatica in my right leg. . . . excruciating pain, at times so intense I nearly collapsed. I can now have a proper bath, . . . sleep in any position, step into my skirts and trousers with ease, put on my tights. I can stoop to fasten my shoes and kneel to weed the garden borders and wash the kitchen floor.
I never drink alcohol, and have ceased taking the anti-inflammatory drugs I was on for the sciatica. I also stopped taking the xxxxxx tablets which I took for pain.'

175

'A few words in appreciation for your introduction to Feverfew . . . it has given me great relief for my rheumatism over the last two years with no side-effects. I have recommended it to several people with the crippling effects of arthritis. These people were amazed as the swelling of fingers etc., disappeared and are now free of pain. I stopped taking them March of this year, until symptoms began again 3 weeks ago. I am now comfortable again and free of pain. I could go on forever about what it has done for me.'

178

'I have been a migraine sufferer for many years, but since taking these tablets I have not had one migraine. I just can't believe it, I have tried so many things in the past.'

179

'I am diabetic and must take xxxxxx tablets and a tiny tablet for water on the lungs. I was taking xxxxx for arthritis but have stopped them now I take Feverfew. The arthritis after several weeks is better. I am 71 (last week) and feel 10 years younger and feel that I can cope with all that must be done in my house and garden. I have completed painting both the ceilings and walls of my lounge and bedroom (high, large rooms) and the windows etc., and will this week start on the ceiling and walls of the small bedroom. Plus tending the back and front gardens and training and walking 3 dogs.'

182

(I think I'm going to try this Feverfew myself. I can't do half what this lady does and I'm only 51. Author)

'I feel I must write and thank you for the information you sent to me three months ago. I have now been taking the tablets for three months.
I have had arthritis since I was 16, I am now 35. First in my knee, then hip, shoulder, but then last year it was very severe in my neck. This has gone progressively worse for two years. The arthritis tablets, of which I tried many did nothing for the pain. The heat treatment eased the pain but a couple of hours later the pain returned.
I had also suffered severe migraine since my second child was born. I had weekly attacks. After three days of taking the tablets the arthritic pain had gone, and I have had not had a migraine attack since. I have never been so free of pain for years. I have told so many fellow sufferers of the value of Feverfew and they have all had excellent results too. The interest in Feverfew is spreading quickly and widely. My aunt in Southport has had excellent results.
I will always be grateful to you, and to the Daily Mail for printing your address. I and fellow sufferers are indebted to you for life. Thank you once again; I do hope that your wife has found alternative relief.'

192

'Dear Mr. Hancock,
Could you please let me have some more leaflets to distribute to my friends who are most interested in Feverfew. I've been taking the tablets for the past 6 weeks, and having previously found it a trial to bus to local towns, I've just returned from a trip to Woking via London, to see a friend. Everyone is amazed as I never go anywhere as a rule.'

200

'Would you please send me another broadsheet on Feverfew as I have passed mine on and it seems to be on tour. As I haven't got it back I have lost the name and address of the Feverfew dealers. I feel so much better I want the world to know.'

201

'Thank you for pamphlets and for finding out about Feverfew's marvellous help re arthritis, as in my own case. I've had arthritis first in 1940 in coccyx of the spine; 4 doctors gave me the news that nothing could be done. . . . then I had what doctors call a frozen left shoulder in 1964,

suffered intense pain, eventually told osteoarthritis and had a plastic shoulder in 1973, told then it was in my spine as well, have been trying every tablet on and off since. As I have been told my bones in my left knee are broken down nothing could be done. The pain I suffered no one knows, and I could not get up and down stairs although I have rails. I told the surgeon at xxxxx hospital that had it not been for my darling dog I would have ended my life. Then I heard of Feverfew, sent off and was amazed at relief, can get up and down stairs and have not bothered about moving downstairs. . . . I'm telling about Feverfew and do realize of course that God has a hand in this also and thank Him every day.
Unfortunately in December 1983 I fell and badly hurt my knee, had 9 injections, no help then I started on Feverfew and "oh boy" could get up and down stairs, pain in knee subsided, and my left hand which was closing began to open more, was to have had an op. on it as I did on the right one but cancelled it. . . . I am 82 but still believe in miracles, with God's help and my faith. Again thank you and may your faith in Feverfew continue to help those who like me believe in trying anything once, and if it helps keep it up.'

208

'Thank you very much for the information about Feverfew. You will be pleased to know that my sister is delighted with the relief from the pain in her hands after taking the tablets. She looks at her hands and says it is a miracle that so much of the swelling has gone down. The times you gave for relief of pain and reduction of swelling were very near. Another blessing is that my sister has found that as the swelling went down, so the feeling came back to the tips of her fingers.'

209

'I was totally cured of migraine (which lasted 7 days at a time) three years ago.'

211

'The Feverfew tablets I have been taking for the past two months have greatly reduced the psoriasis I have had for many months. I have been taking the natural leaf, but the tablet is much better.'

233

'I am writing to thank you for introducing me to Feverfew . . . has completely changed my life.

I had to take early retirement because of arthritis. I used to be a hospital Theatre Porter, and had to give up because of arthritis in my knees. Hospital treatment including shortwave treatment, exercises, drugs and at times having the fluid drained from my knee didn't seem to help much. I was restricted in what I could do but as I have said, Feverfew changed all that.

I can now do decorating, climb steps and all that that entails. Gardening. I can now walk without limping, my knees are no longer swollen. I do not have to put hot water bottles on them to ease the pain. I sleep better and above all I feel better. I have passed on to friends copies of your newsheet. . . Good luck in your venture and once again, thank you.'

235

'. . . . after watching my daughter struggle along with the distressing symptoms (Hayfever) during her attempts in June/July to do her favourite "chore," gardening, I asked her to try the Feverfew. In desperation she did (gardening being her great love) and the outcome was great. It is just on very bad days indeed that she is driven indoors. That in turn prompted me to try it for relief, I hoped, to the many allergic reactions I get to animals, dust, etc., etc., all known irritants in fact, tests have shown. Each time I visit relatives where there are cats or dogs I've been topped up every 4 hours with antihistamine tablets.

This summer I've had to spend a great deal of time over the space of three months at my daughter's, caring for her after an operation . . . so that, deep down inside I dreaded the state I would be in spending all that time where there were three cats. To my utter amazement, and let me say my very grateful thanks, I found that I could get through the day with just one dose of antihistamine.

It was indeed a miracle not to wheeze, fight for breath and these last few years start first of all with a swollen membrane inside my nose, at the back of my throat which was frightening to say the least, as the whole nasal passages seem so swollen it creates this awful panic of what will happen next.

Chance or no, I'm sure we both benefited greatly, maybe this could help others, unless of course it's already a proven fact. Trust this will be of some interest, and will not waste your time or bore you.'

239

'. . . . but to me the great benefit is I don't get "waterworks" trouble. I was taking xxxxxx tablets and after about a year I was getting pain when

I passed water, was going to the toilet approximately every 30 minutes or less . . . I got to the stage where I could not get home from work without leaving a train, going to the toilet and catching the next one, was up 10-14 times each night . . . about then I saw your letter in the Daily Mail and wrote to you to get the information. Within a few weeks my 'waterworks' improved very much, and at the moment although things are not quite back as they were, to me excellent.'

240

'I thought you might be interested to know that before taking the herb I was becoming mildly incontinent—I was having to get up 3 or 4 times each night, which takes about a quarter of an hour and is like doing an assault course—but for the last few weeks I have not had to get up at all.' P.S. It makes me smile when people say in horror "You can't even have a drink at Christmas." What a little price for relief.'

253

'I work in a local hospital as an occupational therapist aide. I see a great deal of arthritis, rheumatoid and otherwise. I had suffered for nearly two years with severe pain in my right wrist and the lower joint of the thumb on that hand.

I found that I was unable to cope with the weight of heavy patients in wheel chairs, and that my hand was very weak. I noticed that my thumb joint had swollen and nodules had appeared. Within a week of taking Feverfew the nodules were disappearing, and the thumb joint began to show its natural shape when bending the thumb, but most of all I am almost free of pain and the strength has returned to my hand.

I have since passed the information on to a nursing sister at the hospital and obtained the tablets for her.'

256

'I have, since I first contacted you in July 1984, as advised taken one Feverfew tablet daily, 2 daily when the pain is bad. The doctor described my illness as a type of arthritis, inflammation of the tendons. . . . one looks around at friends and neighbours, aware how easily other's illness becomes boring.

Feverfew, Ken Hancock, Kathy and Jack Turner = a hand stretched out to help, psychologically invaluable initially, and the mere fact that a harmless herb could help is reassuring after the side-effects of painkillers. After approximately 5 months of using Feverfew I believe this greatly reduces the effects of inflammatory arthritis, works as a lifeline psychologically, in a combination of faith and effect, Feverfew is effective. It seems new sufferers and those with no one to talk to need desperately someone to talk to who understands the shock of one's own doctor, with nothing to offer except painkillers, when coming apart at the seams they need strong support to help them rebuild moral fibre and re-adjust a way of living . . . but it's coming and I'm fighting back now. Ken Hancock, Kathy and Jack Turner and Feverfew have proved invaluable first aid.'

260

'My husband has been taking Feverfew for several months now with excellent results, he is even managing a full-time job after 3 years of virtual disablement.'

264

'I was (and hope I can continue to use that tense) a migraine sufferer for over 20 years. The attacks were frequent and in most cases extremely severe. Twelve weeks ago I started taking Feverfew tablets, one each day first thing in the morning.
For the first 3 weeks although I still had a migraine, the attacks were progressively less severe. Since that time I have been completely clear of any type of headache. I only wish that I had known of Feverfew years ago. I cannot sing its praises too highly. The relief to be able to plan ahead and not to worry that I may be incapacitated at any time by migraine is wonderful. I had reached the stage where even the most powerful painkilling drugs which the doctor could prescribe did not work fully . . . I have not experienced any side-effects.

Nine weeks may not seem a long time to be able to claim a cure but to be without a migraine for one week, for me is a miracle.'

266

'. . . since taking Feverfew (almost 3 months) I'm wondering if it has had an effect on my eyesight . . . having bi-focals and reading glasses as well, now I can do any close work without the reading glasses, and feel so much better generally. I thank you for taking such an interest in your "patients."

274

'I enclose photo of a grateful patient. You asked me to let you know how she got on. At first there did not seem to be any improvement, but we had not realized how bad she was. Her stifles (knees) had given way and become very swollen, then one front shoulder gave way. She could barely move at all. She is a big dog (Great Dane cross), so impossible to lift, and to get her from the lounge to the garden needed a lot of encouragement and 5 or 6 rests. She was in obvious pain, back legs beginning to waste away and we thought she would have to be put to sleep, which broke my heart as she is so gentle and tried so hard to walk for us. So I took her to another vet who x-rayed her and found that she had ankylosing spondylitus (arthritis of the spine), also, causing it to form bone between the vertebrae and eventually become rigid. People and horses get this also. It is very painful whilst ossifying, but once rigid ceases to hurt. This and the knee joints were aggravating each other. He put her on painkillers and eventually xxxxxxx for the swollen knee joint, and hoped she would be O.K. in 6 months. After two months she had improved enough to cut out the morning painkillers, and I then started her on Feverfew. She has literally romped away, and now gets upstairs, and plays and walks quite good distances. She is a mite bandy, cannot run and has to be restrained from leaping about too much, but she is her old happy self and free from pain. her back legs have filled out again where the muscles wasted. I am pleased, as she probably developed this spinal trouble due to terrible beatings as a pup, by her previous owners and I felt that she had suffered enough. She is only 6.'

283

'Thank you for taking the trouble to write to me and advise me on using Feverfew for my arthritic horse. She has been receiving 3 x human dosage for about a month and although she is not yet rideable, she is much improved. I will let you know how she gets on over the winter.'

284

'Having just finished my first bottle of Feverfew. . . . I must write you to say that almost from Day 1 I received relief from arthritis in my left hand.

At the age of 65 and a very keen golfer off a low handicap—you can imagine my absolute despair of a weak grip of the club—over the past few years. I almost gave up the sport.

The rapid improvement has forced me to tell all my business and golfing friends of this wonderful product, and I hope that they obtain the relief that I have. Many thanks and lots of success in the future.'

285

'Just writing to let you know how much better I am on your tablets. A friend at work told me about them. Then she brought me your leaflet to read, and I found out that I wasn't on the right ones. I thought they weren't doing any good. Since I have been taking the right ones I haven't had a migraine, this is since September last year. Every few weeks I had to come home from work as I am a machinist, I just couldn't see. I still can't get the right ones here, but Kath sends them to me very quickly. It's like a miracle for me as I had days off work. I also wear glasses and I have had some leaflets printed for my optician, as he has people who suffer from it.'

323

Feverfew in the news

Feverfew fan club

OVER the years I've written stories of many people who have been helped through ill health by the herb Feverfew.

Recently there have been medical trials which appear to confirm its efficiency and there have been articles about it in the *British Medical Journal* and *The Lancet*.

Because of the huge interest in the herb I'm passing on the address of the non-profit International Feverfew Appreciation Society.

A stamped self-addressed envelope sent to the society at 80 Holbrook Road, Alvaston, Derby, DE2 0DF, will bring you details.

Migraine is the area where many people benefit but there are testimonials at the society that it relieves rheumatism, asthma, high blood pressure and many other complaints.

Healing herb research

I WAS delighted to read your report concerning the research at Nottingham University into the effects of Feverfew in connection with arthritis and migraine.

My own research into the herb began in 1976, and since that time I have answered in excess of 45,000 inquiries. I have also been privileged from time to time to be able to assist in a small way with the work of scientific and medical establishments in the United Kingdom and abroad.

A large number of testimonials—I stopped counting at 1,000—have given a clear insight into the medicinal qualities of the herb, not only in connection with arthritis and migraine but also with psoriasis, stress and a number of ailments related by the factor of stress or trauma, e.g. incontinence and premenstrual tension, a total of 19 to date.

At this point, however, I must stress that a large number of people have been disappointed with the results of the herb simply because they have not been made aware that there are different varieties. Only in a wild variety have I discovered sufficiently reliable qualities, and it is on the use of this variety that my results have been based.

There are, too, other restrictions that apply if satisfaction is to be achieved, and my broadsheet details these. *It is free on application to my home, but please enclose SAE.* To avoid disappointment I must say at this point that I do not sell seeds, plants or tablets.

KEN HANCOCK

80 Holbrook Road,
Alvaston,
Derby DE2 0DF.

Feverfew cures

ARTHRITIS and migraine sufferers are among those who sing the praises of the herb Feverfew.

But it's not just any old Feverfew that is claimed to work wonders in relieving headaches, arthritis and other conditions.

There are four main varieties, and a number of subvarieties: and only one, Wild Feverfew *(Tanacetum parthenium)* is held to have reliable levels of activity. This has to be harvested at the optimum time, and strict attention has to be paid during drying to ensure that the fresh-leaf potency is successfully maintained in the tablet form.

Ken Hancock of Derby has conducted research into Feverfew—largely to try to help alleviate his wife's migraine—for nine years. He says that users include miners who took Feverfew to banish sick headaches caused by working in poor conditions underground. Medieval literature refers to its efficacy in causes of "the worst headache known."

Ken has listed 19 ailments that respond favourably to the herb. These include arthritis, psoriasis and migraine.

For a free broadsheet on his research findings send stamped addressed envelope to Ken Hancock, 80 Holbrook Road, Alvaston, Derby.

Wonder-weed

I WAS delighted to read the letter by Mr. Tier, regarding his relief from the distress of osteoarthritis. Since you published letters from me regarding the use of the herb Feverfew in this connection, testimonials received have opened up new horizons.

My latest research has shown that the herb involves itself, not only with arthritis and migraine, but also with psoriasis and 14 other ailments. This is due to its regulatory effect in one specific area of the body. All the benefits have been recorded as side-effects, while the herb has been taken for quite another reason.

KEN HANCOCK,
Alvaston,
Derby.

Good news

READERS who followed the correspondence in 1984 about the medicinal properties of the herb Feverfew, will be delighted to know that recent articles in *The Lancet* and the *British Medical Journal* have given grounds for optimism. Although official tests have so far been confined to the effects on migraine, benefit has also been noted in arthritis.

My own research has also noted beneficial effects in regard to other stress-related ailments including P.M.T., menopause, incontinence, alopaecia, etc.

There are restrictions which apply to successful use of the herb, and allergic reactions which prospective users should be aware of before commencing treatment. The answers to these and other questions are contained in a free broadsheet available from the address below, but S.A.E. please.

KEN HANCOCK,
International Feverfew Appreciation Society
80 Holbrook Road
Alvaston, Derby
England

The Scientific Confirmation of the Efficacy of Feverfew

The scientific literature on Feverfew, *Tanacetum parthenium*, confirms the long-standing folk usage (especially in England) of the herb for headache, migraine, arthritis and psoriasis.

A full-length study of Feverfew has already been published in England—*FEVERFEW: a traditional herbal remedy for migraine and arthritis*, London, Sheldon Press, 1984, by E. S. Johnson, M.D.

In his book, Dr. Johnson cites a table developed by the University of London computer indicating the proportions of migraine sufferers claiming significant improvement in their condition in terms of frequency, severity or duration of symptoms while taking Feverfew for different periods. *Over 90% of those taking Feverfew daily for 2-5 years indicated significant improvement!* (p. 54)

The scientific literature on Feverfew is as follows:

P.J. Hylands: “Recent studies on feverfew,” *Herbal Review*, 1983;8(3).

Makheja and Bailey: “The active principle in feverfew,” *Lancet*, 1981.

Makheja and Bailey: “A platelet phospholipase inhibitor from the medicinal herb feverfew *(Tanacetum parthenium)*,” *Protaglandins Leukotrienes Med*. 1982; 8, 635.

Heptinstall, White, and Williamson: “Extracts of feverfew inhibit granule secretion in blood platelets and polymorphonuclear leucocytes,” *Lancet*, 1984,i,1071.

Jessup: “Biologically active constituents of *Chrysanthemum parthenium*,” London: University of London, 1982 (Ph.D. thesis).

Bohlmann and Zdero: “Sesquiterpene lactones and other constituents from *Tanacetum parthenium*,” *Phytochemistry*, 1982;21:2543.

Hanington, Jones, and Amess: "Migraine: a platelet disorder," *Lancet*, 1981, ii, 720.

Howe, Fordham: "Polymorphonuclear leucocytes. Origins, functions, and roles in rheumatic diseases." In: Carson, ed., *Immunological Aspects of Rheumatology*. Lancaster, M.T.P. Press, 1981, p. 149.

Berry: "Feverfew faces the future," *Pharmacy Journal*, 1984,222;611.

Johnson, Kadam, Hylands, and Hylands: "Efficacy of feverfew as prophylactic treatment of migraine," *British Medical Journal*, 291, Aug., 1985.

Other Books about Herbs from Keats

Herbs, Health and Astrology by Leon Petulengro
Choosing and Cultivating Herbs by Philippa Back
Growing Herbs as Aromatics by Roy Genders
Making Things with Herbs by Elizabeth Walker
Comfrey by Ben Charles Harris
The Complete Book of Spices by John Heinerman
Eat the Weeds by Ben Charles Harris
Ginseng by Ben Charles Harris
The Guide to Medicinal Plants by Paul Schaunberg and Ferdinand Paris
The Herb Tea Book by Dorothy Hall
How to Make Your Own Herbal Cosmetics by Liz Sanderson
Minnie Muenscher's Herb Cookbook
Secrets of Natural Beauty by Virginia Castleton
The Two-in-One Herb Book by Philippa Back and Alyson Huxley
Way with Herbs Cookbook by Bonnie Fisher
What Herbs Are All About by Jack Challem and Renate Lewin-Challem

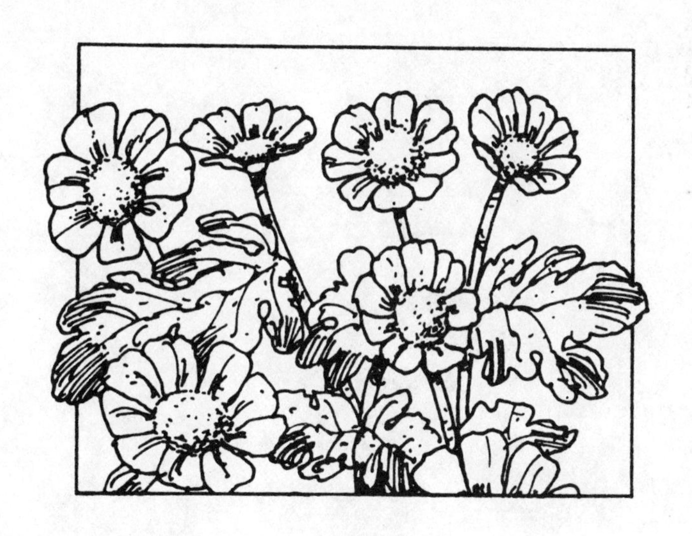

"In the worst headache this herb exceeds whatever else is known."
John Hill, M.D. *The Family Herbal* 1772

A University of London computer analysis found that *over 90%* of those taking Feverfew *(Tanacetum parthenium)* daily for two to five years for migraine experienced *significant improvement.*

TEAR OUT THIS PAGE AND WRITE TO KEN HANCOCK

International Feverfew Appreciation Society
80, Holbrook Road, Alvaston, Derby
DE2 0DF, ENGLAND

Dear Ken Hancock:

Yours truly,

Note: Enclose a self-addressed envelope with an International Reply Coupon which you can buy at the post office.

FEVERFEW

YOUR HEADACHE MAY BE OVER